THE A-Z OF THERAPEUTIC PARENTING PROFESSIONAL COMPANION

Also in the Therapeutic Parenting Books series

Therapeutic Parenting Jumbo Cards
Sarah Naish and Sarah Dillon
Illustrated by Kath Grimshaw
ISBN 978 1 78775 776 9

The Complete Guide to Therapeutic Parenting
A Helpful Guide to the Theory, Research and What It Means for Everyday Life
Jane Mitchell and Sarah Naish
ISBN 978 1 78775 376 1
eISBN 978 1 78775 377 8

The Quick Guide to Therapeutic Parenting
Sarah Naish and Sarah Dillon
ISBN 978 1 78775 357 0
eISBN 978 1 78775 358 7

Therapeutic Parenting Essentials
Moving from Trauma to Trust
Sarah Naish, Sarah Dillon and Jane Mitchell
ISBN 978 1 78775 031 9
eISBN 978 1 78775 032 6

The A–Z of Therapeutic Parenting
Strategies and Solutions
Sarah Naish
ISBN 978 1 78592 376 0
eISBN 978 1 78450 732 9

THE A–Z OF THERAPEUTIC PARENTING

PROFESSIONAL COMPANION

TOOLS FOR PROACTIVE PRACTICE

SARAH NAISH,
SARAH DILLON AND JANE MITCHELL

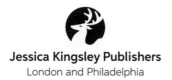

Jessica Kingsley Publishers
London and Philadelphia

First published in Great Britain in 2021 by Jessica Kingsley Publishers
An Hachette Company

1

A CIP catalogue record for this title is available from the British Library and the Library of Congress

ISBN 978 1 78775 693 9
eISBN 978 1 78775 694 6

Printed and bound in Great Britain by Bell & Bain Limited

Jessica Kingsley Publishers' policy is to use papers that are natural, renewable and recyclable
products and made from wood grown in sustainable forests. The logging and manufacturing
processes are expected to conform to the environmental regulations of the country of origin.

Jessica Kingsley Publishers
Carmelite House
50 Victoria Embankment
London EC4Y 0DZ

www.jkp.com

Contents

Introduction   7
Sarah Naish

Part One Drawing the Map: The Trauma Tracker   15
Jane Mitchell

Part Two Building the Cornerstones: The Developmental Foundation Planner . .   53
Sarah Dillon

Part Three Dousing the Sparks: The Behaviour – Assessment of Impact and Resolution Tool (BAIRT).   97
Sarah Naish

Summary: Implications for Practice   141

References   143

Appendix 1: The Trauma Tracker Template   145

Appendix 2: The Developmental Foundation Planner Template   149

Appendix 3: The Behaviour – Assessment of Impact and Resolution Tool (BAIRT) Template   157

Index   169

Introduction

SARAH NAISH

As the author of the bestselling parenting guide *The A–Z of Therapeutic Parenting*, I have been thrilled so see how well the book has been received. I have seen the impact it has made on parents and supporting professionals in being able to understand the fundamentals of developmental trauma and therapeutic parenting. This has resulted in better outcomes for our children and much higher levels of family stability.

This new book, *The A–Z of Therapeutic Parenting Professional Companion*, has been written to complement my parenting guide and provide professionals with guidance and tools to improve their practice and also improve stability for families.

As a former social worker and adopter of five children myself, I still work closely through our consultancy and training company at the Centre of Excellence in Child Trauma (COECT)[1] with fostering and adoption teams. I am always looking at new ways to help social workers and other supporting professionals to be able to build more meaningful, supportive relationships with families. I hope this book goes a long way to achieving that goal.

I am thrilled to have been able to write this book alongside Sarah Dillon and Jane Mitchell, who also work with me at COECT. They bring their own unique perspective.

Sarah is a former child in care, and is now an exceptionally skilled attachment therapist. She works alongside me in training and consultancy. Sarah's work has always been focused on the need to prevent children from having unplanned and damaging moves.

Jane works within our team as an adoptive parent, as our lead 'empathic listener' (the term is explained in the section 'The TRUE model of support and intervention' later in this introduction), and as a trainer. She is excellent at explaining and implementing some of our more complex ideas to parents, and supporting professionals too. Jane has been extraordinarily successful in using her skills to help therapeutic parents to see past difficult behaviours and re-attach to their child.

WHO THIS BOOK IS FOR

Although this book is mainly aimed at supporting professionals, such as social workers and therapists, assisting them to become more skilled and confident about when, and how, to intervene, many skilled therapeutic parents will also be keen to use the tools described. However, it is envisaged that supporting professionals will be using the tools and interventions with practising therapeutic parents, such as foster parents and

---

1   www.coect.co.uk

adopters, although they are also perfectly well formulated to enable and assist with interventions with special guardians and kinship carers.

Some supporting professionals will be working with birth parents too, and the tools contained within this book can be easily adjusted to help support them.

Birth parents with children who have developmental trauma, prenatal stress or underlying conditions are often overlooked. The behaviours arising from these conditions are often prejudged as 'bad parenting' and parents may be sent on 'parenting courses'.

Some parenting courses are effective (such as the SAfE parenting course based on the therapeutic parenting principle[2]; however, parents have told us from their experiences of traditional parenting courses that many are out of date and ineffective for children with trauma. This leads to parents feeling like failures.

Before starting this journey, we strongly recommend you get a copy of *The A–Z of Therapeutic Parenting* (hereinafter called *The A–Z*) and read the first section before you start on this *Companion*. This is because we will be referring to *The A–Z* in relation to all three tools that we introduce in this *Companion*. These will be invaluable to supporting professionals, and by keeping this close identification with *The A–Z*, we are also giving professionals a way to fully utilize the resources contained therein.

WHAT IS THERAPEUTIC PARENTING?

Therapeutic parenting is a deeply nurturing, highly structured parenting style, with a foundation of self-awareness and a central core of mentalization developed from consistent, empathic, insightful responses to a child's distress and behaviours, allowing the child to begin to self-regulate, develop an understanding of their own behaviours and ultimately form secure attachments.

I have explained in *The A–Z* that routines, boundaries, empathy, nurture and self-reflection are essential elements in therapeutic parenting. I often ask parents to imagine that they are holding up a big mirror to their child. Instead of reacting to what the child is doing or saying, they need to reflect back to the child what they think their child's behaviours mean. It is these types of interaction that help to keep the child regulated and able to think more clearly, making links in their own minds about how they think and feel and how they respond.

The other essential element of therapeutic parenting is the need for 'self-care', or rather, 'essential maintenance'. This aspect is often overlooked, or its importance is minimized. If parents do not have 'essential maintenance', they cannot care for their child.

MOVING FROM REACTIVE TO PROACTIVE PRACTICE

When we speak to supporting professionals such as social workers and therapists, they often express feelings of frustration and disillusionment from trying to work within a system that is frequently operating in a *reactive*, rather than a *proactive,* way.

My daughter used to risk her life through a *reactive* philosophy. She would frequently drive her car knowing that one of the tyres was flat or the tracking was off. She was functioning in a reactive way, waiting for the tyre to burst (or be entirely flat) before she would bother to react by going to the garage to get it fixed. This was mainly due to:

- Lack of planning.
- Lack of funds.
- A hope that the problem would magically disappear.
- A belief that if the worst happened, everything would still somehow be okay (hopefully).

Of course, this worked out to be more expensive, and dangerous, as a strategy.

In the UK, as in many other parts of the world, we seem to have adopted a similar approach to caring for vulnerable children.

But children are not tyres.

We are aware that there are many local authorities and agencies working in a reactive manner in adoption and fostering. Although a reactive response can often be due to a lack of knowledge around trauma, there is little doubt that it is also due to an incorrect assumption that it is somehow cheaper to respond to an actual crisis rather than work to prevent one. Some local authorities and agencies are effectively allowing foster parents and adopters to drive about in cars with tyres about to burst.

Many therapeutic parents' experience of reactive planning by their local authority or agency plan is:

- Keep your fingers crossed.
- Remove the child from the family's care (and hope the next family can cope).
- If all else fails, blame the parent.

These types of 'failing to plan' strategies are not only immoral, but they also are costly financially, with further detrimental and hidden costs impacting on:

- The health and wellbeing of the child.
- The mental health of the therapeutic parent.
- The job satisfaction and mental health of practitioners.

My daughter has grown and developed to such a stage where she is now *proactive* around her car. She has realized that taking a low level of preventative action:

- Is more cost-effective.
- Takes less time in the long run.
- Is much safer.
- Is much less expensive.
- Keeps her alive.

Let's all start working in the same way!

HOW TO USE THIS BOOK

This book contains three practical tools that supporting practitioners and parents can use to help them understand and reduce the impact of their children's complex behaviours: **Trauma Tracker**, **Developmental Foundation Planner** and **Behaviour**

– Assessment of Impact and Resolution Tool (BAIRT). Throughout the book we use a composite case history of a *fictional* child called 'Josh' to illustrate these three tools.

In an ideal world, practitioners would use the Trauma Tracker, introduced in Part One, just as a child has been matched with a family, during the moving-in process. The Trauma Tracker is a way of creating an easily accessible record of the chronology of the child – recording their story from conception to coming into care, including any concerns, challenges or disruptions that have occurred.

The Developmental Foundation Planner, introduced in Part Two, can be used in the early days with a child to assess their unmet developmental needs. The planner enables the user to identify specific unmet needs from the information gathered in the Trauma Tracker and from the child's behaviour. These are then addressed by focusing on specific developmental areas necessary for all children. These are referred to as 'cornerstones' and are fundamental to the child's developing attachment to their caregiver.

The BAIRT, introduced in Part Three, can be used at any point with a family where issues arise and behaviours are risking family stability. You will see that in using this tool we refer to 'sparks' (or stressful incidents) being identified where challenges are encountered. These may relate to a behavioural issue and will normally be something that the parent is finding difficult to resolve. Where the parent begins to lose hope, feels out of their depth, or enters compassion fatigue, the stability for the child is threatened. BAIRT offers a quick, structured intervention to stabilize the family, without blame or judgement.

It should be stressed that all three tools can be used separately, on a stand-alone basis. We recommend reading each part of the book and deciding which tool fits best with your practice to help the child you currently have in mind. Even if you are involved with a child who has been in the family for some years, the Trauma Tracker can still be an excellent place to start.

In order to shift supporting professionals from a *reactive* approach to a *proactive* one, some background knowledge and expertise is needed, including:

1. Knowledge of childhood trauma (adverse childhood experiences, ACEs) and the impact this has on the child.
2. Understanding the impact that a child's trauma has on the therapeutic parent.
3. Understanding how therapeutic parenting works.
4. Tools that empower supporting professionals to engage at key moments to prevent problems arising.

As stated above, this resource is most effective used alongside *The A–Z*. In *The A–Z* the first three points are addressed, and are expanded on further in this *Companion*.

For point 4, we provide three easy-to-use tools that are designed to help supporting practitioners cut a path through the complexities of trauma to engage in a meaningful way, ensuring that:

- Children can be kept in families.
- Families can be kept stable and better supported.
- Essential foundations for building secure attachments are put in place.
- There is a dramatic reduction in emergency situations arising along with the associated time allocated.

- The impact of false allegations is significantly reduced, bringing more stability and understanding to these situations.

We have tried and tested the tools extensively and have seen how they have led to a dramatic reduction in family breakdown and unnecessary moves for traumatized children. This was particularly evident within my own (Ofsted 'Outstanding') therapeutic fostering agency, where we used an early version of the BAIRT (see Part Three).

A WORD ABOUT TERMINOLOGY

For many years our training team has been advocating for changes to the terminology widely used in this field. Positive changes are now taking place, and you may notice within this book that there are some terms that have been used very consciously.

'Foster parent', *not* 'foster carer' or 'carer'. We share a fundamental belief that children who have experienced trauma need 're-parenting' or 'therapeutic parenting'. A 'carer' will often finish work and go off shift; a foster parent does not – it is a full-time vocation! In work, I usually use the term 'therapeutic foster parent' to properly describe the professional commitment level of foster parents.

'Therapeutic parent' or 'parent', *not* 'carer'. We use 'therapeutic parent' or 'parent' interchangeably to describe the person with day-to-day care of the child. 'Carer' is not used for the reason outlined above.

'Short breaks', *not* 'respite'. We do not use the word 'respite' to describe a short break or planned sleepover. This is because the definition of the word 'respite' is 'a break from something difficult or unpleasant'. We do not believe our children deserve to be referred to in this way.

'Child', 'traumatized child' or 'child from trauma', *not* 'placement'. We do not use the word 'placement' to describe a child in any circumstance. A family have not had 23 placements – they have looked after 23 children. A child has not had 14 'placements' – they have tried to live and adapt to 14 homes, 14 families, 14 bedrooms and 14 sets of siblings. The word 'placement' dehumanizes the child and minimizes their struggle.

'Children' or 'families', *not* 'cases'. We do not use the term 'cases' to describe children or families; instead, we say 'children' or 'families'. A social worker saying they have '10 cases' is, again, dehumanizing the family.

THE TRUE MODEL OF SUPPORT AND INTERVENTION

Ideally, a truly 'therapeutic' fostering or adoption agency will use the TRUE model of support and intervention when implementing the tools outlined in this book. The key element within this model is to ensure that the parent and child have dedicated 'listeners' and that a skilled attachment therapist has an overview of the whole family.

TRUE stands for:

- Therapeutic
- Re-parenting
- Underpinned by
- Empathy or Experience.

I first introduced the TRUE model in my own (Ofsted 'Outstanding') therapeutic fostering agency in 2010, which was commented on as follows in 2014:

> The service…has developed a therapeutic model of support where up to three workers from the agency support the carer and the children in placement. This has been closely evaluated and received very positively by social workers and child-care professionals. It is excellent practice that is welcomed and highly valued by foster carers.
>
> Local authority commissioners comment very favourably regarding the positive outcomes for children who are placed with carers of the service. For example, one manager stated, 'our children have made exceptional and highly unexpected progress and if all services operated like this one there would be a lot less unplanned endings.'

Since 2010, I have described the TRUE model in my writing and resources and implemented it through training and consultancy in other agencies. I describe the model here in order that readers can easily identify the different roles we refer to throughout the book.

The TRUE model ensures *affective* and *effective* empathy is extended and available to the therapeutic parent, thereby lessening the effects of compassion fatigue and improving stability. The TRUE model relies on *excellent* communication by all parties, indicated by the arrows in Figure 1.

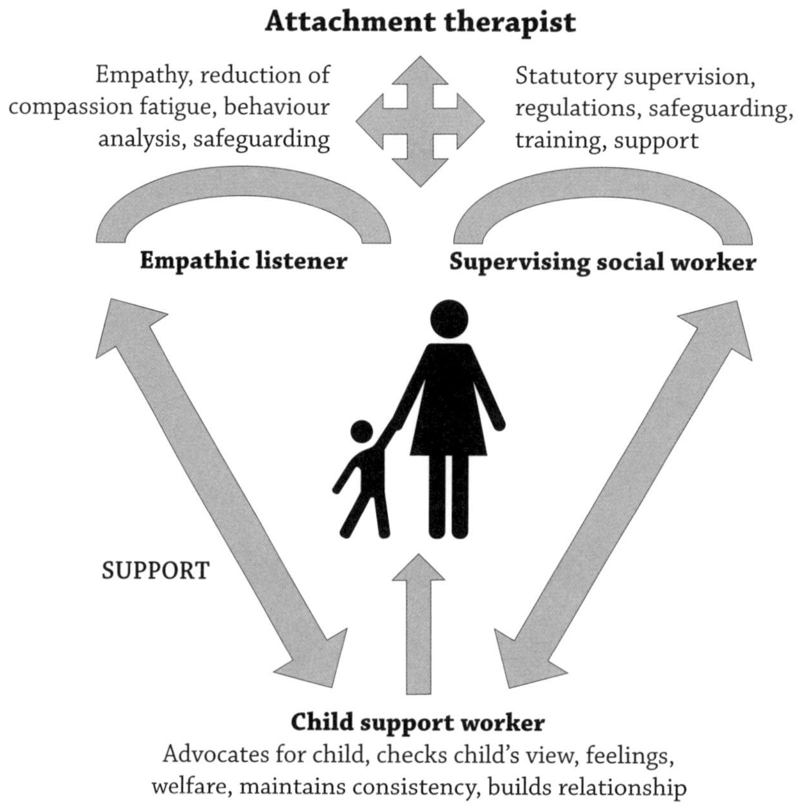

Attachment therapist

Empathy, reduction of compassion fatigue, behaviour analysis, safeguarding

Statutory supervision, regulations, safeguarding, training, support

Empathic listener   **Supervising social worker**

SUPPORT

Child support worker
Advocates for child, checks child's view, feelings, welfare, maintains consistency, builds relationship

Figure 1. The TRUE model

- **Empathic listener:** An empathic listener (or supporter) must be available to the therapeutic parent caring for the child. This must be someone who has had *direct*, personal experience of being a therapeutic parent themselves, preferably over a number of years, and who is familiar with the behaviours and challenges associated with developmental trauma. Specialist mentoring with an empathic ethos, rather than a problem-solving one, enables the therapeutic parent to stay out of compassion fatigue, think clearly and maintain their own levels of empathy for the child. They may also be trained in Dyadic Developmental Psychotherapy (DDP), as developed by Dan Hughes.[3]

  The empathic listener works *alongside* the supervising social worker, and only works directly with the therapeutic parent, not the child. This type of support builds resilience in the therapeutic parent and helps to maintain family stability, reducing the risk of unnecessary and unplanned moves.

  The empathic listener is supervised by a senior attachment worker, usually a therapist or therapeutic social worker, and not by the supervising social worker. This helps to avoid blame and promotes objectivity where there is compassion fatigue. The empathic listener communicates any concerns or safeguarding matters directly to the supervising social worker and child support worker. They keep the rest of the therapeutic team appraised of the therapeutic parent's wellbeing and mental health.

- **Child support worker:** The child support worker will usually be a person with a background in childcare. They may be trained in life story work and Theraplay® and must also have attended training about the impact of developmental trauma on behaviour, therapeutic parenting techniques, managing violent behaviour and compassion fatigue.

  The child support worker is supervised by the supervising social worker and carries out tasks as directed by the supervising social worker. Their role is to support the therapeutic parent on a practical level. This might be through transporting the child to school or family visits. It may also include babysitting, or just being an extra pair of hands at busy times of the day.

  The child support worker has a vital role, ensuring that they represent the child accurately and remain child-focused. This is particularly useful at times where professionals may make assumptions about how the child is feeling.

  The child support worker maintains their relationship with the child and provides consistency. This helps to ameliorate the effects of high levels of change in local authority social workers. They will always visit or phone the child when they go for a short break to another therapeutic parent. The child support worker also communicates concerns directly to the empathic listener where it is felt that the therapeutic parents are showing signs of compassion fatigue or other stress.

- **Supervising social worker:** The supervising social worker is responsible for all legal and statutory obligations being met. They must also be fully trained in therapeutic parenting techniques, developmental trauma and associated behaviours, and the impact on the therapeutic parent. The supervising social worker must be able to judge when empathic listening is required before the

---

3   For more information, see https://ddpnetwork.org

implementation of strategies to manage behaviour. They will be able to support the therapeutic parents in the implementation of these strategies, hold them accountable, and ensure that the child's welfare, emotional progress and attachment is held in central view by the therapeutic team.

The supervising social worker will liaise closely with the empathic listener who is able to work more intensively with the therapeutic parent to help prevent compassion fatigue. They are responsible for supervising the child support worker.

- **Attachment therapist:** The attachment therapist is a DDP (or similarly trained) therapist, with an excellent understanding of developmental trauma and therapeutic parenting.

  The attachment therapist holds TRUE reflection groups with therapeutic parents and associated staff, usually monthly. These groups help to identify patterns and resolve issues before they become problematic. Ideally, a cluster support group of therapeutic parents is established who share an empathic listener, child support worker and supervising social worker. This cluster attends the TRUE groups together, thereby strengthening support and relationships. The attachment therapist supervises the empathic listener.

Over the years, in our training and consultancy, we have been impressed by how some local authorities and agencies have adapted the TRUE model and identified how to fill the key roles from within existing staff, parents and volunteers. For example, some teams have trained up existing mentors to become empathic listeners and social work students have embraced the role of child support worker.

Part One

Drawing the Map: The Trauma Tracker

JANE MITCHELL

The Trauma Tracker collates all the historical information about the child and puts it into one place, so that any emerging behaviours can be seen in the context of the known history of the child.

It can be used to predict possible behaviours as well as giving an understanding of current issues. As such, it can be an essential tool for managing family stability for the therapeutic team, who can then use the information to inform other professionals working with the family.

We use the Trauma Tracker to establish how the history of a child inevitably feeds into the child's behaviours and presentation, and from this we can develop appropriate strategies, have a narrative linking behaviours to the past experience and help parents, professionals and children to work together to create a cohesive team around the family.

WHO CAN USE THIS TOOL?

Any professional who works with children and young people and who has an excellent understanding of the impact of child trauma or adverse childhood experiences (ACEs).

WHAT DOES IT DO?

As mentioned above, the Trauma Tracker sets out the chronology of events in a child's life, and links current presentations to past events to enable behaviours to be managed in a therapeutic way. This generates an environment of understanding and empathy, and moves all those involved with the child away from blame-based responses. We have seen increased stability in all of our families as a result of this tool combined with a therapeutic approach.

WHO DOES IT HELP?

The family and the child, who can be much more effectively supported; the professionals involved, as they can see more clearly the challenges faced by the parents and child alike; and any agencies involved, as the team around the child can work more effectively.

Below is an example of a blank Trauma Tracker. I will explain the process of filling it out as we move through this part, with a completed example given at the end for Josh.

Child's name: **Date of birth:**

History/ chronology	In utero/birth	Antenatal	Known significant events/dates
History of family moves			
Symptoms of trauma			
Current issues			
Event			
Links to history			
Strategies			

History/ chronology	In utero/birth	Antenatal	Known significant events/dates

BACKGROUND

The Trauma Tracker is the brainchild of Sarah Dillon, and came about as a result of her experiences of working with foster families and seeing how an absence of knowledge about a child's history creates huge problems for the child, the parents, and for those supporting the family. Sarah came to see me in December 2018 with a template and I then took the idea forward.

For reasons of confidentiality we are not able to share the specifics of the young people Sarah worked with, but below we have created one fictional case history to explain the kinds of issues that the Trauma Tracker can help to address.

Example case history: CATHERINE

A child, Catherine, was living with the family of a very experienced single foster mum, Penny.

Catherine was very hard to look after and connect with as she could fly off the handle easily and was very clingy and attention seeking (Naish 2018, p.261). With the help of the empathic listener and the attachment therapist, Catherine was just beginning to settle. Penny told the empathic listener how she found Catherine happily lying on her tummy, playing with toys like the other children. This was a breakthrough!

Then one day Catherine got to school feeling upset. She was unsettled all day. She did not want to get on the bus. The school phoned Penny, who took 45 minutes to reach her through traffic and arrived to find that the school had called social services because Catherine had alleged that her mother had hit her. She was taken immediately to an alternative foster parent.

The attachment therapist and empathic listener worked together to find out what had happened.

It transpired that Catherine was very scared as one of her **birth** parents had recently come out of prison and she thought that they might come and find her – stressor no. 1.

Catherine got on the school bus and thought she saw one of her siblings – stressor no. 2.

As she walked down the bus, one of the children, who reminded her of another of her siblings, bullied and hit her – stressor no. 3.

She worried about the home journey all the way through her school day and got into trouble for not paying attention – stressor no. 4.

She was so scared that she refused to get on the school bus, which made her worried that her foster mum would be angry with her – stressor no. 5.

It took a long time for Penny to get to school to pick Catherine up, and Catherine thought she would be in big trouble. The stress was so huge that she got muddled with her memory, remembering how she used to be hit for 'being a nuisance', and so she said to the teachers, 'My mum hit me!!' The teachers assumed that she meant Penny. Catherine was not returned home.

Had there been a Trauma Tracker in place, this history could have been pieced together and Catherine may either not have been removed or she may have been returned to Penny. This breakdown of the family when she was just settling would have been highly detrimental to Catherine.

The shift from reactive to proactive practice

So the Trauma Tracker is primarily about using the child's history to inform our responses and to shape our initial understanding of the child. This knowledge is essential for supportive professionals who wish to shift their practice from reactive to proactive.

By increasing our knowledge of the child's experience we can work out how to support the child using strategies such as empathy (respecting the child's perspective as their truth and bearing witness to their emotional pain), empathic commentary (demonstrating understanding of the difficulties the child is facing in the here and now, see the examples given in *The A–Z* [Naish 2018, p.45]) and 'naming the need' (where the attuned parent is able to interpret and verbalize the child's inner world; examples given in *The A–Z* [Naish 2018, p.57]).

The Trauma Tracker helps us to trace back behaviours to their underlying causes. Most of the challenging behaviours that we see are rooted in fear and insecurity, and occur as a direct result of the child's observation, experience or unendurable shame and fear. This includes behaviours that are violent, either physically or verbally aggressive, or rejecting. Many parents and supporting professionals believe that violence and aggression is a result of anger, when the root emotion is actually *fear*.

Fear is the trigger for a survival response that is entirely unconscious. The threat to survival (which can be something as seemingly trivial as a hunger pain) causes the amygdala to fire, and sufficient activation of the amygdala causes the fight or flight response. The child who is violent or aggressive is showing their survival response, and by unpicking their early experience we are able to clearly understand the anxiety that provoked the reaction.

If we create a Trauma Tracker as soon as we are able to, preferably as part of the transfer process that brings a child into an organization or service, we can start to predict from the outset what unresolved issues may present, and can fully support the therapeutic parent to help the child move past their trauma.

It may sound unlikely that, to use a common example, a hunger pain can cause a meltdown of epic proportions, but remember that this is something frequently experienced by children who have been neglected and left hungry, or who have had unpredictable access to food. We have heard stories of children chewing on their cots in their hunger, going through bins, eating rubbish off the floor. If this has been your child's experience, then the pain of hunger will bring the memory to the forefront, creating panic that is very real.

Part of the role of the Trauma Tracker is therefore to enable us to access our empathy for the child and experience horror at what they have endured in their short lives.

Understanding the impact of trauma

In the course of my work I speak to literally hundreds of families. I have noticed that there are times when parents (biological, adopted, foster, kinship or other – they are all parents!) and professionals will say something like 'They had a little bit of trauma' or even 'They did not have any trauma – they were picked up from hospital by a lovely foster family and then we adopted.' Let's be clear here – there is no such thing as 'a little bit' of trauma.

RELEVANCE OF PRE-BIRTH (IN UTERO) EXPERIENCE

Sometimes we find that in utero experience is ignored, despite this having an impact on the developing child. For example, a confirmed and registered addict will not stop her habit during pregnancy and then start again after birth. If we know that the mother suffered an addiction, we can be sure that there will be repercussions – the evidence for this lies in the development and behaviour of the child, and this has been observed on numerous occasions by the authors of this book.

DEVELOPMENTAL STAGES

Below, I outline a series of developmental stages that are helpful to keep in mind when considering the impact of the child's history and the way that this has affected their physical, cognitive, social and emotional developmental areas.

The architecture of the brain – where it starts

The way that children (and adults) interact with and understand the world is dependent on their experiences, and the crucial period of time for this growing perception of self, others and the world is during the earliest developmental phase of the brain – from conception to around two years old.

Pre-birth experience

EMBRYO STAGE: UP TO WEEK 9

During this stage the embryo is formed of three layers of cells. The first of these layers, the ectoderm, has cells that will differentiate to become skin, the nervous system and connective tissue. The spinal cord and brain originate from a neural groove that is formed in this layer of cells. The middle layer of cells, the mesoderm, is differentiated to form bones, muscles, kidneys and the reproductive system. The final layer of cells, the endoderm, differentiates to form lungs, intestines and the bladder.

This means that, from the first weeks of life, the embryo is already developing the structures and vital organs that will determine health after birth. From around 10 weeks the mother and embryo share a circulatory system, which means that they are also sharing hormones, nutrients and any medicines that the mother ingests.

Clearly if the mother is drinking alcohol, smoking or abusing narcotics, the embryo's undeveloped systems will be affected by these toxic substances with a range of effects that will impact on future development. The baby's systems are simply not sufficiently developed to deal with these toxins.

We already know that damage to physical development can occur in this early stage – for example, spina bifida and cleft palate. We also know that smoking while pregnant will affect the growth of a baby. Alcohol, narcotics or high cortisol levels have unseen effects, which are covered in more detail below.

FOETAL STAGE, WEEK 9 ONWARDS

Because the mother and child have a shared system, there is a connection between them. The foetus is able to hear and is subjected to the emotional state of the mother because of her hormones that are directly passed to the foetus through the shared circulatory system.

Sue Gerhardt (2004, p.67) explains, 'As early as pregnancy, the stress response is already forming within the developing foetus and can be affected by the mother's state of health. In particular, her high cortisol could pass through the placenta into his brain.'

The development of the digestive, reproductive, musculo-skeletal and nervous systems of the foetus also depend on the mother's ability to provide adequate nutrition as the placenta continues to grow and create a circulatory system connecting mother and child. This is why there is a great deal of support available to pregnant women to ensure the health of both mother and child.

The foetus develops quickly, and importantly some aspects of foetal development seem to be triggered by their in utero environment to prepare them for the outside world. For instance, being exposed to high levels of cortisol in pregnancy is then linked to high levels of cortisol (the primary stress hormone) in the baby, which then persists after birth.

The relevance of this to the Trauma Tracker is that it is important to remember that maternal illness, mental health, level of nutrition and level of stress can all have a developmental effect before the baby is even born.

The baby may have neonatal abstinence syndrome (NAS) as a result of opioid addiction (they are born addicted and suffering withdrawal) or the baby may have developmental issues as a result of foetal alcohol syndrome (FAS) due to the mother's excessive consumption of alcohol. Smoking compromises respiratory systems and means that the baby is likely to have a low birth weight.

Mothers who are looking forward to birth connect with their developing baby very quickly and are intensely interested in tracking the development of their baby, flooding their system and the baby's with dopamine and oxytocin (the happy hormones). This is very positive for the baby to have low levels of stress. However, the reverse is true when the baby is flooded with cortisol, which has a detrimental effect on neurological development.

Why is this important? Because in order to start unpicking the trauma that a child has suffered, we have to go back to the very beginning.

Children from trauma will present with a range of diagnoses and behaviours. This is quite bewildering and can be non-productive because sometimes there is little or nothing in the way of practical strategies offered (although sometimes it can be useful to have a diagnosis in order to access support).

Sarah Naish (2018) suggests that if we stop attempting to diagnose and look instead at the historical facts and the presenting behaviours, we will invariably find answers to the underlying cause of the child's challenging behaviours, which are, in fact, the strategies that the child has adopted to cope with their overwhelming experiences.

Below is another fictional case example, this time to illustrate the significance of pre-birth experience.

Example case history: SANDRA

Sandra is the adoptive parent of a little boy I shall call Simon. Sandra called me because she was struggling with his need for control and violent outbursts.

Sandra was told how lucky she was to have this little boy because he had gone from hospital to foster parents and was then adopted quite quickly. However, she simply could not understand the behaviours she was seeing and had difficulty accessing help. Unfortunately, many of the professionals working with the family were blaming her parenting.

I asked what she knew about Simon's history, and learned that Simon's mother was a registered addict, and that as a result he was born addicted. His body and brain had to try to grow and develop whilst being subjected to heroin, and he was born into the pain of an enforced withdrawal.

It is also likely that his mother had high cortisol levels. Addicts have hard lives – chaotic and stressful, often associated with violence – which typically lead to high cortisol levels that impact on the baby, with Simon having high cortisol levels triggered in utero. When Simon was born and had to endure withdrawal, no one was there to comfort, reassure or regulate him. He must have been terrified.

Simon also had the trauma of separation and rejection from his birth mum. Then, his earliest days were spent alone, in a hospital cot.

He was subsequently moved into a caring foster home that delivered him to an adoptive family at age 10 months.

When Simon got older and realized his friends all lived with their birth mums, and saw babies being born and kept, and loved, and valued, it made him wonder what it was about him that was so bad that his own mother didn't want him?

His earliest days have given him lifelong issues. Talking Simon's history through with me helped his adoptive mum to regain her empathy, and I was able to validate many of the decisions that she made instinctively, such as maintaining contact with Simon's initial foster family. Sandra is now learning about therapeutic parenting, and we're hopeful that this will be a turning point for her and for Simon.

The thing I really like about the Trauma Tracker is that it enables us to read between the lines, and puts the child at the centre, as do the other two tools in this book. We do not dehumanize children by calling them 'placements' and we validate their awful experiences. We allow their behaviour to tell us the story of what happened to them, and to do this we are open to the fact that they have had awful experiences pre-birth and after.

Early childhood development

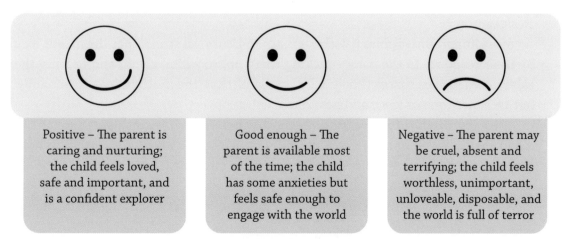

Positive – The parent is caring and nurturing; the child feels loved, safe and important, and is a confident explorer

Good enough – The parent is available most of the time; the child has some anxieties but feels safe enough to engage with the world

Negative – The parent may be cruel, absent and terrifying; the child feels worthless, unimportant, unloveable, disposable, and the world is full of terror

Figure 2. Different types of parenting

The relationship between a caring adult and a child has a huge impact on the development of babies and young children.

Sue Gerhardt (2004, p.38) notes that, 'without the appropriate one-to-one social experience with a caring adult, the baby's orbito-frontal cortex is unlikely to develop well'. She goes on to describe how the mutual enjoyment of the relationship is one of the ways to ensure that this happens.

In an ideal world, a baby has a parent who is able to maintain their attunement with the baby's needs. Indeed, because of early bonding in utero, the parent may already feel that they 'know' this child, and, understanding their vulnerability and fragility, are fiercely protective of their new-born infant.

The first few weeks are often an intensive and challenging time while the parent and child work out how to manage this new dynamic. The baby learns that they can influence the parent, and the parent learns that they can soothe and regulate the child, who then learns to trust the parent. What is learned initially within the small family unit is then extended to include carefully chosen others, such as grandparents, and then to the wider community as the baby matures.

What many people forget is that in these earliest days the baby's experiences form the architecture of their brain – their understanding of the world and how to deal with it. Daniel Siegel (2015, p.22) confirms how neural pathways are activated: '…more common, everyday experiences…shape brain structure. The brain's development is in part an "experience-dependent" process, in which experience activates certain pathways in the brain.'

In addition, during this time the parent is 'potentiating' the baby's skills and abilities (enabling the baby to make the fullest use possible of these).

Babies are born with the ability to see (unless they are visually impaired), but the development of sight is mediated by the parent stimulating vision with bright toys and drawing the baby's attention to objects.

Although babies have a skeletal system, muscles and motor neurones, the ability to master these body parts is mediated by the parent, or relationally mediated. For example, a parent helps their baby to coordinate and control their body by playing with them and encouraging them to explore intentional movement, perhaps by giving them a toy to reach for.

Babies have sensations that the parent helps them to interpret and respond to – whether it be hunger, cold, loneliness, boredom or tiredness. The parent will often do this with a running commentary about their thoughts: 'I wonder if you are hungry?'; 'It is time for lunch now!'; 'I can see you are getting tired. I am here. Let's just help you to sleep now.'

Most importantly babies have huge fears and 'survival stress' that the parent regulates by their response to the baby – picking them up, soothing them, and helping them to calm down. Sue Gerhardt (2004, p.23) explains that 'the mother does this mainly with her face, her tone of voice and her touch'.

The baby also has survival needs – food, water, safety, warmth and a sense of being loved – which the parent meets. Whether or not a baby's needs are met, their brain will respond to their survival need and they will adapt their behaviours to whatever they need to do in order to stay alive.

A child whose needs are met will have a sense of safety, and engage in exploration and learning.

A child whose needs have not been met will have great difficulty in managing their engagement with the world.

Sue Gerhardt offers the example of a child named 'Genie' who suffered the most awful neglect and was not introduced to the world outside until the age of 13. Genie showed global developmental delay in her physical, emotional and cognitive development (Gerhardt 2004).

The baby whose needs are met learns to trust the adult. They are curious and want to explore. They know that their parent is always there to keep them safe. They know that they can engage their parent's attention, claim a cuddle or receive a smile.

They also start to experience the emotional pain of a 'relationship rupture', such as earning their parent's disapproval if they do something that is dangerous or socially unacceptable.

This typically happens once they enter toddler stage when their ability to crawl, toddle and reach for objects can cause a parent to react in a way the baby finds distressing. For example, a baby who has just learned to crawl discovers that they can also climb stairs. The parent reacts out of fear by shouting at them to stop, which scares the baby. The baby then cries – they feel a rupture in their close relationship with the parent. The parent then makes the hazard safe by blocking the stairs, and is able to cuddle and calm the baby, restoring the baby's emotional equilibrium.

This is what we term a 'relationship repair' – essentially, how we 'make up' after a quarrel, allowing for resilience and trust that the relationship can withstand a few bumps.

A baby whose needs have not been met, or whose needs have been inconsistently met, leads to the development of a negative internal working model, as previously discussed. The above forms the basis of the internal working model (also see p.25 *The A–Z* 'The child's internal working model'). They do not develop a 'template' of how to engage positively with the world. They do not learn that adults can be trusted. They may learn ways to manage the terror of their existence according to the situation they are in. They may need to learn to be quiet and invisible, to run away and hide, or to fight, shout or scream for attention. *Any* attention will do. Whatever the situation, these children learn to be constantly alert for danger – scanning their surroundings and hypersensitive to body language and sensory signals from the world around them. They notice the smallest changes and can interpret these as indications of impending doom.

More detail about how childhood trauma affects behavioural responses may be found in Chapter 1 of *The A–Z* (Naish 2018, pp.18–28).

THERAPEUTIC PARENTING AND THE TRAUMA TRACKER

There is a lot of divided opinion about therapeutic parenting – this is often from parents, but it can also come from professionals, sometimes because of a system that is in place (in schools, for example, with reward systems or inappropriate unrelated sanctions) or because therapeutic parenting is misunderstood (for example, use of natural consequences can be seen as letting children 'get away with it', and using repair and reconciliation can be seen as 'rewarding a child for bad behaviour').

This is not true. We do not shame children, but we let them know that we understand 'why' they behaved the way they did. We support them to change without judgement or blame. We support parents to be the best parents they can be using empathy, validation, strategies and essential tools. We support professionals to support parents and children. The overall structure is empathic and supportive and seeks to ask 'why?' rather than throw blame.

Here's another fictionalized case history that shows how knowledge and understanding of the early life not only of the child, but in this case of the parent too, can inform an intervention that changes families' lives.

Case history example: MOHAMMAD AND YUSUF

Mohammad is a single parent looking after his nephew Yusuf under a Kinship Care Order.

Mohammad had not experienced good parenting himself, and was very triggered by Yusuf. Yusuf was in his early teens and was big and heavy, throwing his weight around – using controlling threatening behaviours and swearing to get his own way.

This was understandably very difficult for Mohammad, who felt that he should have respect and that Yusuf should not get away with such behaviour; he was also upset at being physically hurt. Mohammad signed up for some one-to-one sessions with the National Association of Therapeutic Parents, and we started to talk about his own childhood.

It became apparent that Mohammad needed to help himself to work through some of the memories of his own childhood experiences before he could help Yusuf, so he had some Delta Touch Therapy, a therapeutic intervention that enables a client to de-link past trauma using a touch technique with a qualified therapist.[1] This helped him to see his challenges more clearly and to separate his own issues from Yusuf's.

Mohammad started taking charge of his own responses. He did not rise to challenges, and stepped out of conflict. Sometimes he left notes reminding Yusuf of things that needed to be done, but he did not insist on them being done or pick a fight.

Gradually, a change happened. Yusuf started (sometimes) bringing his plates down after eating, and (sometimes) emptied the dishwasher. The shouting and swearing stopped. Their relationship improved. The incidents of violence were fewer and further between.

Mohammad found it so hard, but he could see the changes and persevered. He used narratives (conversations developed with the help of our therapeutic team) to help Yusuf to link his behaviours to his early experiences. He reminded Yusuf that he was safe in the family.

This took months and is ongoing, but the spiral towards a family breakdown has turned into a positive process, building trust and respect.

FALSE ALLEGATIONS

In addition to helping us to understand the needs of children and the support needed by families, the Trauma Tracker can be a useful tool to help resolve false allegations. False allegations can happen when memories of historic trauma are triggered by sensory input, which activates the firing of the amygdala and the fight or flight response.

For the child suffering from developmental trauma with intrinsic memories of abuse, this can mean their experience of specific sensory triggers will immediately activate their

---

1   For more information on this, visit www.thehavenparentingandwellbeingcentre.com

amygdala and mediate a fight or flight response, which will feel as though it is happening in the present. Daniel Siegel explains:

> ...repeated experiences of terror and fear can be engrained within the circuits of the brain as states of mind. With chronic occurrence, these states can become more readily activated (retrieved) in the future, so that they become characteristic traits of the individual. In this way, our lives can become shaped by implicit memory, which lack a sense of something being recalled. We simply enter these engrained states and experience them as the reality of our present experience. (Siegel 2015, p.55)

This leads to challenge, as professionals need to take allegations at face value because safeguarding principles have to be observed and allegations must be investigated.

What we are suggesting is that having a clear understanding of the history of the child can provide more context to such investigations. The Trauma Tracker may provide information that helps to make sense of the allegations – for example, historical evidence of any previous allegations, a clear history of events and a way to show how events have led up to an allegation that is actually a triggered trauma memory.

In such cases, if there is no evidence, and if parents' recording of the child's experiences in logs or diaries is clear, the child need not face the disruption and further erosion of self-esteem of being removed from their family.

Understanding how memory operates is not simple, however. Siegel (2015) explains that what we commonly understand as memory – that is, conscious and narrative, involving recall of events within a time frame, and a way of remembering important facts, dates, etc. – falls short of explaining its complexity. Memory actually involves the integration of sensory input and enables us to make sense of our past, understand our present and anticipate our future (or consequences): 'memory is the way past events affect future function' (Siegel 2015, p.46).

This may be *explicit* memory – fully 'remembered' facts, events and sensations – or *implicit* memory – based on experiences we cannot recall consciously.

This is the basis of the internal working model, as discussed: 'Our earliest experiences shape our ways of behaving, including patterns of relating to others, without our ability to recall when these first learning experiences occurred' (Siegel 2015, p.47).

The physiological response to a survival threat (the fight or flight response) is the secretion of stress hormones such as cortisol and noradrenaline. Cortisol may stop or reduce explicit processing by blocking the functioning of the hippocampus (part of the limbic system of the brain that is necessary for long-term memory and recall), while noradrenaline increases implicit encoding. The stress response can prevent a fully retrievable explicit memory being encoded, but the sensory and contextual triggers (shouting, an expression, a smell, a place, time of year) will be implicitly encoded and can provoke a further stress response on an unconscious level.

For the child suffering from developmental trauma with memories of abuse, this can mean that specific sensory triggers will immediately activate their amygdala and mediate a fight or flight response that will feel as though it is happening in the present.

I have developed an analogy for this. Imagine you are filing some papers – this stands for encoding memories in your hippocampus.

The items you are filing are date stamped, sequential and in a system that allows them to be retrieved (this is your day-to-day experience of encoding memory in your explicit memory). Suddenly there is a major incident, and the fire alarm goes off (a trauma occurs, and your amygdala fires, which sends the hippocampus offline).

Unable to remember how to file, you stuff all the papers in the safe (implicit memory) and run. Later, after the event, you cannot remember what you did with those files – they are not accessible.

However, the next time the fire alarm goes off, the implicit memory is once again triggered and you retrieve the information.

The significance of this for children in care is that sensory data that is imperceptible to others may literally cause them to feel that they are back in the situation of trauma, and this will be exacerbated when the child has high circulating cortisol due to stress such as approaching an anniversary (for instance, of a move or transition, birthday, Christmas, anniversary of a traumatic event). In that moment, a fleeting facial expression, a sound, a smell or an action may be misinterpreted.

The child remembers the incident but experiences it in the present and makes a disclosure such as 'My mum hits me'. However, the child may be referring to a historic incident, which may or may not be previously known. The child is confusing what *happened* with what is *happening*.

For example, I remember a parent telling me how her dysregulated adopted son threw a milk carton, flipping it over. (Dysregulated means a child who has lost the ability to keep control of their big feelings and who is beginning to behave in challenging ways.) She reached out to catch the milk carton to prevent a spillage. He misinterpreted this as a hostile gesture and accused her of hitting him. She was dumbfounded, but unfortunately he was triggered into a violent episode.

If there had been a Trauma Tracker for this child, it could have been established that there had been physical abuse, and the parent could have been warned about keeping her hands neutral when the child was dysregulated and giving him tools to help him understand his own reactions (see Parts Two and Three).

Fully understanding trauma and helping a child to heal is, of course, a *process* and not an *event*. It requires skill, empathy and a team of supporting professionals around the family to get it right.

The Trauma Tracker is an essential tool to help supporting professionals to be proactive and effective in their approach. In relation to false allegations, it allows them to both predict possible triggers and respond to the associated behaviours appropriately.

This should lead to greater stability within families and better outcomes for children. Taking a *reactive* stance means that you are always firefighting. By being *proactive* we can create real changes for the better and alleviate the strain on the resources of social services.

AN OVERVIEW OF THE TRAUMA TRACKER

The Trauma Tracker initially takes all of the known history and chronology possible about the child, from their in utero experience (if known) up until the time the Trauma Tracker is filled in. This may include birth family history, place in family, lifestyle, when known to social services, date of care order, other court dates, and any foster families the child has lived with, including reasons for any disruptions and any other known traumatic events. This is all vital information.

Consider a child who has had 98 moves in two years (and I have met a child who has experienced this). How on earth can that poor child begin to make sense of themselves or of the world?

In the world of social work, this might be given the minimizing description of 'The child has had 98 placements', language that could infer that the number of placements are the child's fault – 'they are *so* difficult'. On reading this, anyone new to working with the child and their family may not feel that the family will succeed – the parent is concerned at the level of behaviour they may be facing, and the child *knows* that they will be moved on.

The reality behind the very short statement above is that, with an average of one move every two weeks, this child has had:

- 98 sets of parents.
- 98 sets of siblings.
- 98 different bedrooms.
- 98 different sets of rules.
- Multiple ruptures in friendships.
- Multiple schools.
- Multiple social workers.
- Multiple therapists.

From historic information and a chronology, we can form a good idea of the child's internal working model – their representation of themselves, the adults in their life and the world.

This is the way the child views themselves, which depends on an attuned relationship with a protective parent – the parent; the parent's attitude to the child and their response to them shows the child a view of themselves (for more on this, see Naish 2018, pp.25–26).

When using the Trauma Tracker, always remember to consider the detail of the lived experience of the child, and how they will have experienced it.

USEFUL APPLICATIONS

Anticipate triggers

The Trauma Tracker helps us to identify potential triggers. By having a clear chronology including dates, we can let the foster parent know that the child may feel more 'wobbly' around these dates.

If, for example, the child was removed from their family in February, we might see their anxiety, expressed as challenging behaviours, begin to emerge around a week before the event. We can help both the parent and child by giving them a narrative to explain this, saying something like: 'I can see you are finding things hard at the moment. It was about this time of year that you left your birth family. That must have been so hard for you – do you want to talk about that? Remember, you are *not* leaving here and we are keeping you safe.'

Many children have huge difficulty with Christmas – there are so many additional triggers involved, such as lights, smells and sounds and songs. For some children all these triggers reactivate trauma memories.

Anniversaries of any kind are hard to manage. Having a timeline helps us to plan ahead and be prepared.

The Trauma Tracker helps us to understand the child's presentation by giving us a lens through which we can predict the child's behaviours. Behaviours can be explained by past events. If there was a history of a chaotic lifestyle, possibly including neglect and being left alone, the child will have no sense of predictability and reliability, so they will panic when they are hungry or if they cannot see you.

If they have witnessed or been subject to domestic violence they will believe that you control people by attacking them. If they have been subjected to sexual abuse they will replay these behaviours with adults, children, toys or by drawing.

Encourage understanding

Children recreate what is familiar – if the place they felt safe was their dirty, smelly bedroom, with broken toys and bedclothes smelling of urine, they can unconsciously try to recreate that chaos in the foster, adopted or other parent's home.

Parents need to be helped to understand and gently support the child through the huge changes they are going through. Using the Trauma Tracker in this way can prevent family breakdowns and the child having to move in an unplanned way. This also enables us to understand false allegations by providing a context, again preventing an unplanned and traumatic move for the child and intense trauma for the foster parent.

It is also important to remember that moves will cause regression and reinforce a negative view of self. Where a child is moving on from a family it is vital to explain to the new parent that this may be expected, and to give them tools and strategies to manage.

I have spoken to many foster parents who told me how the children were lovely for a week or two and then started to show their 'true' selves. Of course, what actually happened was that the child began to experience safety and then started showing the foster parent their trauma through their behaviour.

With the Trauma Tracker this can be managed in a very different way by 'naming the need' and being empathic about the child's past experiences. By using the Trauma Tracker in this way, we can create stable and safe environments for our families. Of course there will be difficulties and 'bumps in the road', but as the adult grows more confident in their ability to help the child, the child grows confident in the security of the family unit, and will then start to invest in the relationship, leading to a shift in their behaviours.

The Trauma Tracker is very useful in explaining the behaviour that 'comes out of nowhere', as it helps parents and professionals to unpick the behaviours and find the root cause. Children get overwhelmed quickly, and we need to understand that a child who has lived with violence, abuse, addiction or chaos, or the child who has been scapegoated in their own home, singled out for neglect, abusive language and subjected to rage and disproportionate abuse and punishment from their parent, will be hypersensitive to the mood of the parent and become very fearful. Building the parent's understanding of this can reduce or prevent scapegoating and blaming the child, which effectively replicates their early experience.

Support difficult transitions

Because events are noted as they occur and added to the Trauma Tracker it helps us to identify the critical time when a child is experiencing a burgeoning attachment to their parent.

This creates a paradox for the child because they experience feelings of betrayal, fear (many children are told of dire consequences if they talk) and extreme vulnerability. The child wants to trust, but to do so feels so scary and makes them feel vulnerable. The child typically starts showing 'push-me-pull-you' behaviour – they approach and then avoid. They come for a cuddle and then inexplicably pinch or hit.

This is a time when the family needs increased support to manage the behaviours and address the underlying fear. Maybe the parent might say something like: 'I know what's happening. You are scared to trust me in case I decide to send you away. That is not going to happen.' I remember this happening to a brilliant foster parent I know. Her child would snuggle up to her in the mornings, and then, after a while, would suddenly start really attacking her. I explained what I thought was happening and we discussed how to manage this by cutting short the cuddle *before* the child's fear of rejection took over. The family are still together.

Make the Trauma Tracker work for you and the families you support

To conclude, the Trauma Tracker gives professionals a step-by-step process to unpick the child's history and to use it to better inform their own practice and ensure that there is support around the family, especially around the time that the child transitions into the family and when any stressful incidents (which we call 'sparks') arise that may compromise the stability of the family.

PUTTING STRUCTURES IN PLACE BEFORE YOU START

The Trauma Tracker can help when we are first settling a child as we will be able to identify where the child has severe trauma, but generally speaking, we absolutely know that there are some essential structures that we need to have in place around a child to help them. These are outlined in more detail in Chapter 3 of *The A–Z* (Naish 2018, p.32), but briefly, they are:

Establish a strong routine: This gives consistency, predictability and reliability, and increases the child's sense of being held in a strong structure that keeps them safe and ensures their needs are met.

Establish yourself as the 'unassailable safe base': This does *not* imply that you engage in battles for control and dominancy. It means that you are a constant presence for the child on good days and bad, and that if you say a thing will happen, then it does: 'The skilled therapeutic parent needs to be in control, even though we are establishing control through empathic and nurturing methods' (Naish 2018, p.124).

Honesty: '...it is vital to say what you mean and mean what you say' (Naish 2018, p.35), and this is because children from trauma are absolutely tuned into our body language. If your body language does not match up with what you are saying, it triggers all their fears and creates distrust. This, in turn, leads to adverse behaviours. It is also a mistake to think we can protect a child from information about what has happened to them. They were there. They may not be able to readily access the memory and 'remember' because the trauma was so great that they were forced to encode the experience as an intrinsic memory, held as an emotional trigger against future occurrences. If your trauma was caused by the very people or person you are reliant on for survival, and are still dependent on, this causes a terrible conflict. Under these circumstances the stress hormones can cause the memory to be encoded differently to give the child a chance of survival (see the earlier discussion on false allegations).

Have strong, clear boundaries: Again, this is not about picking battles to control children. It is about consistency. For example, if the TV gets turned off at 8 pm, the parent does not give in to the requests for '5 minutes more'. They might instead check beforehand when the programme finishes in case they need to record it to watch later. If the child is upset about this, the parent is empathic, but firm. Likewise, even if the child or children seem to be having fun and coping and the parent is tempted to give them extra time for the activity as a result, the therapeutic parent will remember that the boundary between fun and overwhelm is a fine line indeed, and will stick to their original plan.

Sarah Dillon and Sarah Naish write about the essential therapeutic parenting input and therapeutic parenting strategies that should be applied in Parts Two and Three of this book.

FILLING IN THE TRAUMA TRACKER – JOSH

As mentioned in the 'Introduction', we use the fictional character of Josh and the team around him throughout this book to help explain and explore all three intervention tools. Josh is a composite child based on several children we have worked with, and all identifying characteristics have been changed.

The following is the basic, unpopulated Trauma Tracker before it is filled in with all the information we have about Josh. As you can see, I have added examples and reminders to the blank sheet to help to prompt the social worker or professional as they fill out the form.

Child's name: **Date of birth:**

History/chronology	**In utero/birth (e.g. domestic violence, drug/alcohol addiction; mental health, illness, birth trauma, premature, maternal illness, abandoned)**	**Antenatal (e.g. abuse, domestic violence, drug/ alcohol addiction, family known to social services; unavailable mother – mental health, addictions, hospitalizations)**	Known significant events/dates (e.g. hospitalizations, bereavement, date of removal from family, separation from siblings)

History of family moves (e.g. moves in and out of foster care; kinship care; number of moves, attempted reunification; dates of moves between families)

Symptoms of trauma (e.g. generalized anxiety, self-harm, aggression and violence; demand avoidant; stealing, lying, nonsense chatter, attention needing; sexualized behaviours)

Current issues

Event

Links to history

Strategies

History/chronology

So what do we know? The following is the history that we have at the time of our subject child's move into the current foster care agency in 2016.

Josh came to live with Linda at the age of four years, six months. We know that he has a younger and an older sibling. The family were known to children's services from when Josh was one year of age, due to concerns raised by the health visitor, the nursery and the school of the older child as a result of the presentation of the children and the house during school time and when the health visitor came to check on the latest sibling.[2]

Children's services monitored the family for a few months, and it was believed that the mother had managed to take the advice and support on board and so the case was closed. It was subsequently re-opened due to a call to the duty social worker in March 2014, and the children were subject to a Child Protection Plan in April 2014 and a Pre-Proceedings Meeting in May 2015 due to evidence of domestic violence within the home, substance abuse and neglect.

Josh was placed with an emergency foster parent for a night after the children had been left home alone, and he then went to live with his great aunt. This was not a long-term plan as there were concerns about her ability to care for Josh due to her own health issues. In July 2015 Josh went to live with his first foster family.

A full Care Order was granted the following year. During September 2016 the foster parent who was a single woman gave notice due to Josh's escalating behaviours – hitting her and swearing at her and the other children in the household. Josh also disclosed that he had been left at home alone and had no food when he was living with his birth parents. His behaviours at school were also escalating.

In October 2016 Josh was moved to a new foster agency where the TRUE model (Therapeutic Re-parenting Underpinned by Empathy or Experience), devised by Sarah Naish, was implemented (for a reminder, see the 'Introduction'). Josh went to live with a single foster parent, Linda. It was at this point that the empathic listener filled in the Trauma Tracker at the request of the attachment therapist. We can immediately pick out the history/chronology from the case notes:

2   'Presentation' refers to the way the house and the children looked on observation. For example:
House: Clean? Tidy enough? Food available? Bedding? Toilet rolls? Towels? No excrement from pets, etc.?
Children: Clean? Tidy? Clothes fit and are appropriate for age and weather conditions? Children appear happy and relaxed or subdued? Engaging or withdrawn? Excessive fighting/swearing, etc.?

Child's name: Josh Williams   **Date of birth:** 14 December 2012

History/chronology	In utero/birth (e.g. domestic violence, drug/alcohol addiction; mental health, illness, birth trauma, premature, maternal illness, abandoned)	Antenatal (e.g. abuse, domestic violence, drug/alcohol addiction, family known to social services; unavailable mother – mental health, addictions, hospitalizations)	Known significant events/dates (e.g. hospitalizations, bereavement, date of removal from family, separation from siblings)
November 2013: family came to notice of children's services 2014: Child Protection Plan 2015: Pre-Proceedings Meeting May 2015: emergency foster care for one night after being left home alone May 2015: went to live with maternal great aunt; concerns due to her health issues July 2015: Interim Care Order granted; moves into foster family no. 1 October 2016: moves into Linda's care			

History of family moves (e.g. moves in and out of foster care; kinship care; number of moves, attempted reunification; dates of moves between families)

Symptoms of trauma (e.g. generalized anxiety, self-harm, aggression and violence; demand avoidant; stealing, lying, nonsense chatter, attention needing; sexualized behaviours)

Current issues

Event

Links to history

Strategies

In utero/birth and antenatal

As we know that severe concerns were raised at the Pre-Proceedings Meeting about domestic violence, substance abuse and neglect, we are also able to add in some possibilities for pre- and post-birth trauma – as a result of the domestic violence there is a high possibility of high circulating cortisol.

There is no way of knowing whether the birth mum was regularly using alcohol or recreational drugs during pregnancy, but this is a possibility. Failing to record these details about the mother's lifestyle can mean that we miss significant issues for the child as they grow and develop. The importance of this information is that it would give us a more complete picture about what has happened to Josh, and we can trace from this the impact on him and the effect it has on his behaviour.

It is important for the social worker to gather as much information as possible, including any disclosures that have been unsubstantiated, because this may help us to understand any behaviours that emerge later. The social worker can work with the attachment therapist to get a full understanding of the implications of the historical events. This will help with preparation and getting a structure in place.

If we fill in these two columns, we can then begin to clarify our understanding of Josh.

Child's name: Josh Williams   **Date of birth:** 14 December 2012

History/chronology	In utero/birth (e.g. domestic violence, drug/alcohol addiction; mental health, illness, birth trauma, premature, maternal illness, abandoned)	Antenatal (e.g. abuse, domestic violence, drug/ alcohol addiction, family known to social services; unavailable mother – mental health, addictions, hospitalizations)	Known significant events/dates (e.g. hospitalizations, bereavement, date of removal from family, separation from siblings)
November 2013: family came to notice of children's services 2014: Child Protection Plan 2015: Pre-Proceedings Meeting May 2015: emergency foster care for one night after being left home alone May 2015: went to live with maternal great aunt; concerns due to her health issues July 2015: Interim Care Order granted; moves into foster family no. 1 October 2016: moves into Linda's care	Exposure to domestic violence – likelihood of high circulating cortisol	Domestic violence – this may mean increased circulating cortisol Josh has disclosed that his father touched him and that he was left alone and left hungry	

History of family moves (e.g. moves in and out of foster care; kinship care; number of moves, attempted reunification; dates of moves between families)

Symptoms of trauma (e.g. generalized anxiety, self-harm, aggression and violence; demand avoidant; stealing, lying, nonsense chatter, attention needing; sexualized behaviours)

Current issues

Event

Links to history

Strategies

We know that there has been domestic violence that Josh may have been subjected to or that he may have witnessed, or both. We know that high circulating cortisol will mean that Josh is very reactive to stressful situations – because he already has high levels of cortisol, it is easy for him to be overwhelmed by additional stressors. He has disclosed that his father touched him inappropriately, and although this is unsubstantiated, this should be recorded in case he is involved in sexualized incidents or makes further disclosures.

He has also been increasingly violent towards family members and increasingly unmanageable at school. This indicates that he is feeling very unsafe, both in home and the school environment. It does *not* indicate that he is just a 'naughty' child.

Sarah Dillon sometimes says 'safety comes in, trauma comes out'. The meaning of this is that when Josh began to be established in a safe environment, he then started 'showing' the foster parent his trauma. Some of the trauma happened at a pre-verbal stage and was so traumatic that his body retained this as an intrinsic memory, as discussed earlier.

Josh only had words for some of his experiences – some were too traumatic and had to be demonstrated when the memories emerged. So he showed violence and hit out, especially at the single female foster parent and her children. This is behaviour he had observed in his daily life. Because this was not a therapeutic parenting fostering agency, the foster parent was not given the tools she needed to try and manage this in a therapeutic way, and so the situation became uncontrollable.

Known significant events/dates

We can also fill in the known significant dates, and these can be added to over time. Significant dates such as birthdays, anniversaries of moves between families, hospitalizations, accidents or known traumatic events give us a way to predict when stress levels are likely to increase through the year, and enable us to plan the support that will be necessary for the family.

The importance of this information gathering is that children hold an intrinsic memory – when an anniversary is coming up of a significant event, it can trigger some of their trauma for them. If we have a record of possible dates, we can use this information to plan or to be prepared. Once we add the dates, the Trauma Tracker looks like this:

Child's name: Josh Williams   **Date of birth:** 14 December 2012

History/chronology	In utero/birth (e.g. domestic violence, drug/alcohol addiction; mental health, illness, birth trauma, premature, maternal illness, abandoned)	Antenatal (e.g. abuse, domestic violence, drug/alcohol addiction, family known to social services; unavailable mother – mental health, addictions, hospitalizations)	Known significant events/dates (e.g. hospitalizations, bereavement, date of removal from family, separation from siblings)
November 2013: family came to notice of children's services	Exposure to domestic violence – likelihood of high circulating cortisol	Domestic violence – this may mean increased circulating cortisol	December: his birthday, Christmas
2014: Child Protection Plan			May 2015: removal from family; first moved into foster home for a night; went to live with great aunt
2015: Pre-Proceedings Meeting		Josh has disclosed that his father touched him and that he was left alone and left hungry	July 2015: moved to foster home no. 2
May 2015: emergency foster care for one night after being left home alone			October 2016: moved to foster home no. 3 (Linda)
May 2015: went to live with maternal great aunt; concerns due to her health issues			
July 2015: Interim Care Order granted; moves into foster family no. 1			
October 2016: moves into Linda's care			

History of family moves (e.g. moves in and out of foster care; kinship care; number of moves, attempted reunification; dates of moves between families)

Symptoms of trauma (e.g. generalized anxiety, self-harm, aggression and violence; demand avoidant; stealing, lying, nonsense chatter, attention needing; sexualized behaviours)

Current issues

Event

Links to history

Strategies

Unfortunately, the information we have been given does not tell us when he was separated from his siblings, but this is likely to have been around or before July 2015.

What this information tells us is that he may be particularly vulnerable in December due to his birthday, and also because of the overwhelming nature of Christmas. Children from trauma often have a tension whereby they ask for loads of things to prove that a parent loves them. Because they have not had an attuned relationship, their empty feeling has to be filled with 'things' that replace the regulation and soothing of a responsive parent. This might mean many presents, lots of food, sweets or other items that can stand in for a secure attachment figure. It is not uncommon for these things to then be destroyed as the child feels that they do not deserve to have anything nice due to their internal working model.

Christmas is, of course, overwhelming to most children, but there may be specific trauma attached to this if children have lived with a truly chaotic lifestyle, such as is indicated by Josh's history. For instance, another child in care that I know of who came from a background where there was drug misuse and multiple moves found a person dead from an overdose on the sofa on Christmas morning. I find that it is very hard for adults to begin to imagine these sorts of situations and the profound and long-lasting effects they produce – but we must keep this in mind (see 'Sabotaging' in The A–Z [Naish 2018, p.244]).

We have a duty to help the child to explore and make sense of these terrible events so that they can move away from the terrible shame and sense of responsibility they carry.

In addition, Josh may have trauma memories that emerge in May, July or October due to the fact that these are the months that his moves between families occurred. This information can be held and noted in case of any emergence of linked behaviours around those times. This would be likely to be rejecting or self-isolating behaviours; fear of rejection expressed as criticism of the foster parent; or even running away or self-harming.

History of family moves

Looking at the history of family moves will tell us a great deal about Josh's ability to feel that he deserves a place in a family or a home. We do not know whether Josh moved around a lot as a child, but having a chaotic lifestyle can often involve multiple moves to avoid debt or to avoid the law or social services. What we do know is that he had at least four moves between families by the time he was four years old:

1. Family home to emergency foster parent.
2. Foster parent no. 1 to great aunt.
3. Great aunt to foster parent no. 2.
4. Foster parent no. 2 to foster parent no. 3 (Linda).

This is important because these multiple moves in a short space of time serve to highlight to the child that they are 'bad', that they are 'not wanted'. Children are egocentric and therefore believe that everything is their fault anyway, and children from trauma live in shame because they believe they brought all these terrible things down on their own head.

In Josh's case, from his point of view, his own mother did not keep him. His own dad hurt him. His great aunt did not want to keep him. Foster parent no. 1 moved him on because she could not manage his adaptive behaviours – she did not have the knowledge to understand or the skills to help him make the necessary links with his past.

Based on these experiences Josh has an expectation of what will happen next. He is 'very bad' so nobody will want him, especially when they get to know him. He expects future rejection and loss.

It is, of course, easy for any of you reading this book to say that I do not know this, and that I am making big leaps here based on very little evidence, but the behaviour speaks for itself. It is my firm belief that, rather than always giving the parents the benefit of the doubt, we should instead give children the benefit of the doubt. A child is born in innocence. They then have to find a way to understand the world and how to survive in it. Children are not innately evil – but they can be moulded into terrible forms by their experiences.

Sometimes (fortunately, very rarely) we do come across child murderers – but they were not born killers. Somewhere along the line they did not get the basic lessons of right and wrong; they did not learn empathy; they were shown no compassion. We depend on our parents for development of these most human of traits. If our parents are unable to provide us with a template for kindness and being mindful of others, how and where is this ability able to be developed?

If the child has a parent who accepts them with their history and behaviours and starts working in a therapeutic way, this developmental gap can be filled and the effects of the original abuse can be diminished.

We will now add in the family moves to our Trauma Tracker, which is already yielding a lot of information:

Child's name: Josh Williams   **Date of birth:** 14 December 2012

History/chronology	In utero/birth (e.g. domestic violence, drug/alcohol addiction; mental health, illness, birth trauma, premature, maternal illness, abandoned)	Antenatal (e.g. abuse, domestic violence, drug/alcohol addiction, family known to social services; unavailable mother – mental health, addictions, hospitalizations)	Known significant events/dates (e.g. hospitalizations, bereavement, date of removal from family, separation from siblings)
November 2013: family came to notice of children's services

2014: Child Protection Plan

2015: Pre-Proceedings Meeting

May 2015: emergency foster care for one night after being left home alone

May 2015: went to live with maternal great aunt; concerns due to her health issues

July 2015: Interim Care Order granted; moves into foster family no. 1

October 2016: moves into Linda's care | Exposure to domestic violence – likelihood of high circulating cortisol | Domestic violence – this may mean increased circulating cortisol

Josh has disclosed that his father touched him and that he was left alone and left hungry | December: his birthday, Christmas

May 2015: removal from family; first move into foster home for a night; went to live with great aunt

July 2015: moves to foster home no. 2

October 2016: moves to foster home no. 3 (Linda) |

History of family moves (e.g. moves in and out of foster care; kinship care; number of moves, attempted reunification; dates of moves between families)

1. Family home to emergency foster parent no. 1, May 2015
2. Foster parent no. 1 to great aunt, May 2015
3. Great aunt to foster parent no. 2, July 2015
4. Foster parent no. 2 to foster parent no. 3 (Linda), October 2016

Symptoms of trauma (e.g. generalized anxiety, self-harm, aggression and violence; demand avoidant; stealing, lying, nonsense chatter, attention needing; sexualized behaviours)

Current issues

Event

Links to history

Strategies

By adding in the year that the moves occurred, we can see that at age three Josh had three moves in one year as well as the removal from his family and the only home he had known. By age four he had moved again.

It is absolutely vital for us to pause and consider how this felt to such a young child. His whole world was changed. He was moved, meaning a new house, new family, new expectations and new rules. He was probably moved with no explanation of what was happening or any attempt to make sense of it for him. And then back to familiarity – there is at least a link to family with his great aunt – although he was then moved on again.

How was this explained to him, I wonder? Was he told he could not stay because of his behaviour? Because he was too much trouble, too active? Maybe he was told his great aunt loved him but could not keep him.

In this case there is further proof that people who love you reject you. The only link is himself – it must be his fault. Then no sooner does he start to settle down and feel safe, his trauma memories start to emerge in his behaviour. He can't keep his feelings in. Before you know it, he is moved again.

I would like you to pause and consider the experiences that this very young boy has had by the age of four. Who is helping him? Although he had play therapy, it was not consistent, seemingly, and was not continued as part of his care plan moving on. So who is helping him with this huge burden?

Symptoms of trauma

Next, we will consider what his symptoms are, how he is presenting at the time the Trauma Tracker is written:

Child's name: Josh Williams **Date of birth:** 14 December 2012

History/chronology	In utero/birth (e.g. domestic violence, drug/alcohol addiction; mental health, illness, birth trauma, premature, maternal illness, abandoned)	Antenatal (e.g. abuse, domestic violence, drug/alcohol addiction, family known to social services; unavailable mother – mental health, addictions, hospitalizations)	Known significant events/dates (e.g. hospitalizations, bereavement, date of removal from family, separation from siblings)
November 2013: family came to notice of children's services 2014: Child Protection Plan 2015: Pre-Proceedings Meeting May 2015: emergency foster care for one night after being left home alone May 2015: went to live with maternal great aunt; concerns due to her health issues July 2015: Interim Care Order granted; moves into foster family no. 1 October 2016: moves into Linda's care	Exposure to domestic violence – likelihood of high circulating cortisol	Domestic violence – this may mean increased circulating cortisol Josh has disclosed that his father touched him and that he was left alone and left hungry	December: his birthday, Christmas May 2015: removal from family; first move into foster home for a night; went to live with great aunt July 2015: moves to foster home no. 2 October 2016: moves to foster home no. 3 (Linda)

History of family moves (e.g. moves in and out of foster care; kinship care; number of moves, attempted reunification; dates of moves between families)

1. Family home to emergency foster parent no. 1, May 2015
2. Foster parent no. 1 to great aunt, May 2015
3. Great aunt to foster parent no. 2, July 2015
4. Foster parent no. 2 to foster parent no. 3 (Linda), October 2016

Symptoms of trauma (e.g. generalized anxiety, self-harm, aggression and violence; demand avoidant; stealing, lying, nonsense chatter, attention needing; sexualized behaviours)

Aggression and violence; some sexualized language (mild); incidents of sexualized behaviour. Inability to manage school with overwhelmed violence and aggression. Showing signs of jealousy of Linda's grandchild

Josh has a great deal of superficial charm and quickly 'befriends' people

Current issues

Event

Links to history

Strategies

Looking at this alongside the information we have already used to complete the Trauma Tracker so far, it is easy to link the behaviours to his past and to be able to see how very scared Josh must be.

Josh has a great deal of superficial charm, and this seems to create the impression that everything is fine; however, the additional behaviours show that this is far from the case. What Josh shows us with his charm is that he is terrified of adults and has an absolute need to make friends with them. If they are his friends, maybe they won't hurt him – he will be as friendly as he needs to be to stay safe.

Unfortunately, it is extremely likely that up until the point of Josh entering the therapeutic parenting agency that no one thought about how to 'join the dots' for Josh. There is a prevalent view that very young children who lack the vocabulary to explain what has happened to them will not remember because they are too young. Sadly, this does not fit with our knowledge of how understanding and sense of self is created. We do not remember terrible trauma in great detail – because we have to survive. However, intrinsic memories are subconscious and sensory in nature, as we have discussed.

Sensory triggers act like switches alerting our systems to danger, safety, comfort, pain, and so on. Our body holds these associations – and this is well known on an everyday level. Is there a scent, taste, place, smell or sound that instantly reminds you of a person or a time in your life? Is this something that is a lovely memory or something you choose to ignore? Do you seek this out or do you avoid it?

Another prevalent misconception is that we should not upset the child by reminding them of things. If only it were this simple! We cannot protect a child from what has already happened to them. They were there. They remember. They may not have a narrative to give you, but small things will remind them, and they will show you with their behaviours and actions. It is very important to let the child know that you are aware of what has happened and that it was not their fault. In Josh's case we make this link very clear for him, as you will see later.

Josh is also showing some signs of jealousy about Linda's grandson Tom, who is two. The grandchild is a direct rival for Linda's attention, and as such is a threat to Josh's survival. No doubt this seems to be farfetched; however, Josh has no sense of being able to trust adults, and so anyone taking Linda's attention from him when she is the source of everything he needs to survive is a major threat to him. This is *not* conscious; it is part of the way his central nervous system and limbic area are interpreting his stress, and this can only happen based on previous experience.

Current issues

This section of the Trauma Tracker deals with the most current issues that are presenting so that we can work out a therapeutic approach:

Child's name: Josh Williams   **Date of birth:** 14 December 2012

History/chronology	In utero/birth (e.g. domestic violence, drug/alcohol addiction; mental health, illness, birth trauma, premature, maternal illness, abandoned)	Antenatal (e.g. abuse, domestic violence, drug/alcohol addiction, family known to social services; unavailable mother – mental health, addictions, hospitalizations)	Known significant events/dates (e.g. hospitalizations, bereavement, date of removal from family, separation from siblings)
November 2013: family came to notice of children's services 2014: Child Protection Plan 2015: Pre-Proceedings Meeting May 2015: emergency foster care for one night after being left home alone May 2015: went to live with maternal great aunt; concerns due to her health issues July 2015: Interim Care Order granted; moves into foster family no. 1 October 2016: moves into Linda's care	Exposure to domestic violence – likelihood of high circulating cortisol	Domestic violence – this may mean increased circulating cortisol Josh has disclosed that his father touched him and that he was left alone and left hungry	December: his birthday, Christmas May 2015: removal from family; first move into foster home for a night; went to live with great aunt July 2015: moves to foster home no. 2 October 2016: moves to foster home no. 3 (Linda)

History of family moves (e.g. moves in and out of foster care; kinship care; number of moves, attempted reunification; dates of moves between families)

1. Family home to emergency foster parent no. 1, May 2015
2. Foster parent no. 1 to great aunt, May 2015
3. Great aunt to foster parent no. 2, July 2015
4. Foster parent no. 2 to foster parent no. 3 (Linda), October 2016

Symptoms of trauma (e.g. generalized anxiety, self-harm, aggression and violence; demand avoidant; stealing, lying, nonsense chatter, attention needing; sexualized behaviours)

Aggression and violence; some sexualized language (mild); incidents of sexualized behaviour. Inability to manage school with overwhelmed violence and aggression. Showing signs of jealousy of Linda's grandchild
Josh has a great deal of superficial charm and quickly 'befriends' people

Current issues

October 2016: Josh has had multiple moves between families. Josh is presenting with a developmental age of two emotionally. Josh is developing strong feelings for Linda. This has caused a fragile attachment. Josh is having extremely violent episodes and targeting Linda. When he calms down he seeks comfort and proximity. Josh has suffered significant domestic and possible sexual abuse in the past and over a period of time. Josh has also been swearing – 'Fuck off, you bitch!' – calling Linda a 'bitch' and a 'bad mum'. He also refers to his or others' genitals a lot as 'nuts'. This behaviour is showing us trauma that he has witnessed

Event

Links to history

Strategies

Josh's multiple moves mean that he has no trust in his place in any family being permanent. He is showing behaviours more usual for a two-year-old in his lashing out and tantrums. Of course, the difficulty is that this is bewildering for the foster parent because of his actual age of four, and this is a very common issue where misunderstandings can arise.

We have seen that many supporting professionals will talk about children showing a younger developmental age without understanding how this can be dealt with by simply adopting a response that is suitable for the emotional age of the child. There may be significant differences in physical, social, emotional and cognitive development, each of which may need a different response appropriate to the developmental stage that the child is exhibiting (Sarah Dillon explains experiential age in Part Two). Because of what he has observed and experienced, Josh has seen and heard things that are inappropriate for his age.

When he is upset and angry, these actions and words resurface due to the triggering of intrinsic memory, hence the swearing and violence. In addition, Josh has had repeated experiences of rejection, and it is very often the case that the child who is fearful of being rejected will start using rejecting behaviours towards their parent as a form of self-defence.

With regard to the aggression that Josh is showing, this is related to the domestic violence that he observed. When he was tiny, he was powerless to defend himself, and he had to avoid being the subject of violence by being very charming and friendly.

Josh has seen that strong men use their power to hurt women and children. If he is going to survive, he needs to be strong and powerful too. It is all too common for parents who are subjected to child-to-parent violence to be blamed and judged for this – supporting professionals will often tell them that they are not setting firm enough boundaries for the child, that they are allowing these behaviours. These professionals have clearly never been in proximity with a child who is in a defensive rage as a result of an overactive amygdala. Once the fight or flight response is initiated, the child is fighting for their life. They are fired with adrenaline that is ensuring that their heart is pounding harder, their heartbeat is raised and their lungs are working to oxygenate blood that will enable muscles to be ready to fight or run. At this point, the thinking brain is not online – when you are about to die, you need to act, not think. The child in this state is immensely strong – they can really cause damage. I know of a foster son aged nine who was able to pull a radiator off the wall when in a state of overwhelm. That's extreme – but not unusual.

Some supporting professionals will want to examine each incident minutely to identify a trigger. Unfortunately, because of the high levels of stress experienced by children from trauma, the trigger can be a kind of 'last straw' effect – they may have been able to just about maintain regulation all day (at school, for instance) and then, as soon as they are asked to do something else (like hang their coat up), they explode.

There will also be historical triggers and events, which is why we need to look carefully at anniversaries, birthdays and the chronology to establish when trauma occurred. Aggression can be lessened in a number of ways, such as 'naming the need', giving an empathic commentary, ensuring that there is structure and routine, and that changes are kept to a minimum as well as by using the additional tools outlined in this book.

Finally, Josh is showing intense jealousy of Linda's grandchild. Although when they are apart Josh thinks of him, wants to buy him sweets and asks to see him, when the grandson is actually there, Josh can quickly become very angry and stressed, lashing out at Linda. He needs support to name the need – that nothing bad will happen, that there is enough of Linda to go around, that we can care for more than one person at a time – but this will take time and repetition.

This completes the historical part of the Trauma Tracker that is useful to refer back to so that all professionals supporting the family can remember what has happened to create the situations that occur.

Significant events

The next part of the Trauma Tracker is to record significant events so that these can be dealt with using supportive tools:

Child's name: Josh Williams   **Date of birth:** 14 December 2012

History/chronology	In utero/birth (e.g. domestic violence, drug/alcohol addiction; mental health, illness, birth trauma, premature, maternal illness, abandoned)	Antenatal (e.g. abuse, domestic violence, drug/alcohol addiction, family known to social services; unavailable mother – mental health, addictions, hospitalizations)	Known significant events/dates (e.g. hospitalizations, bereavement, date of removal from family, separation from siblings)
November 2013: family came to notice of children's services 2014: Child Protection Plan 2015: Pre-Proceedings Meeting May 2015: emergency foster care for one night after being left home alone May 2015: went to live with maternal great aunt; concerns due to her health issues July 2015: Interim Care Order granted; moves into foster family no. 1 October 2016: moves into Linda's care	Exposure to domestic violence – likelihood of high circulating cortisol	Domestic violence – this may mean increased circulating cortisol Josh has disclosed that his father touched him and that he was left alone and left hungry	December: his birthday, Christmas May 2015: removal from family; first move into foster home for a night; went to live with great aunt July 2015: moves to foster home no. 2 October 2016: moves to foster home no. 3 (Linda)

History of family moves (e.g. moves in and out of foster care; kinship care; number of moves, attempted reunification; dates of moves between families)

1. Family home to emergency foster parent no. 1, May 2015
2. Foster parent no. 1 to great aunt, May 2015
3. Great aunt to foster parent no. 2, July 2015
4. Foster parent no. 2 to foster parent no. 3 (Linda), October 2016

Symptoms of trauma (e.g. generalized anxiety, self-harm, aggression and violence; demand avoidant; stealing, lying, nonsense chatter, attention needing; sexualized behaviours)

Aggression and violence; some sexualized language (mild); incidents of sexualized behaviour. Inability to manage school with overwhelmed violence and aggression. Showing signs of jealousy of Linda's grandchild
Josh has a great deal of superficial charm and quickly 'befriends' people

Current issues

October 2016: Josh has had multiple moves between families. Josh is presenting with a developmental age of two emotionally. Josh is developing strong feelings for Linda. This has caused a fragile attachment. Josh is having extremely violent episodes and targeting Linda. When he calms down he seeks comfort and proximity. Josh has suffered significant domestic and possible sexual abuse in the past and over a period of time. Josh has also been swearing – 'Fuck off, you bitch!' – calling Linda a 'bitch' and a 'bad mum'. He also refers to his or others' genitals a lot as 'nuts'. This behaviour is showing us trauma that he has witnessed

> **Event**
>
> 15 November 2016: Josh and Linda were feeding the ducks and had some stale bread. Josh did not want to share. He called Linda names. His behaviour escalated, leading to him making demands for lunch and beginning to hurt Linda. He continued to escalate, punching Linda's face, shouting 'Fuck off, you bitch', also shouting that Linda should be nice to him as he had a bad time when he was little – punching and headbutting. A man who was in the area intervened, asking if everything was okay. Josh calmed down sufficiently to allow Linda to get him home. Unfortunately Josh dysregulated when he got home, and broke Linda's grandson's little chair. He carried on punching, kicking and headbutting. Linda supported Josh to go upstairs, but he headbutted and kicked her. Josh then began to calm. He stated he did not want to be angry any more and was fine. Josh later reveals that he sometimes wants to die, and discloses that his father tried to suffocate him with a blanket after Josh tried to get between his mum and dad during an argument. He also disclosed that a younger sibling was there too
>
> **Links to history**
>
>
>
> **Strategies**

Here we can see the escalating behaviour. Josh has had a trauma memory resurface, which has caused him to completely lose control. This may be due to timing as he had a move around the same time of year, or it may be that something about the man who intervened reminded him of his father. This was a significant incident, partly in its severity and partly because of the subsequent disclosure that gives a clearer understanding of what Josh has been through.

This is vital to our understanding of his behaviour and gives us further links to his history. Because Linda is a female single parent, for example, Josh finds it hard to believe she can keep him safe. He is scared and angry and lashes out using the words he remembers from his birth home. He breaks possessions (a chair and toys) of the grandson, who represents a survival threat to him. Once he has allowed himself to be regulated, he makes his disclosure – it is fresh in his mind.

Links to history

This allows us to make the links back to his history in the Trauma Tracker. It also shows us where his extreme levels of anxiety originate – trying to reconcile the person who should keep you safe with the person who literally tried to kill you is a really intense situation that causes disassociation. It also explains some of his jealousy – he tried to protect his family, and his father tried to kill him. This means that Linda's grandson Tom represents a secondary threat because Josh's need to protect the smaller child places him in a life-threatening situation, and therefore the young child is a threat in two ways: first, because of the historical event, and second, because of his need to monopolize his foster mum. Having the historical information to hand makes it easy to start putting the pieces together.

Child's name: Josh Williams   **Date of birth:** 14 December 2012

History/chronology	In utero/birth (e.g. domestic violence, drug/alcohol addiction; mental health, illness, birth trauma, premature, maternal illness, abandoned)	Antenatal (e.g. abuse, domestic violence, drug/alcohol addiction, family known to social services; unavailable mother – mental health, addictions, hospitalizations)	Known significant events/dates (e.g. hospitalizations, bereavement, date of removal from family, separation from siblings)
November 2013: family came to notice of children's services 2014: Child Protection Plan 2015: Pre-Proceedings Meeting May 2015: emergency foster care for one night after being left home alone May 2015: went to live with maternal great aunt; concerns due to her health issues July 2015: Interim Care Order granted; moves into foster family no. 1 October 2016: moves into Linda's care	Exposure to domestic violence – likelihood of high circulating cortisol	Domestic violence – this may mean increased circulating cortisol Josh has disclosed that his father touched him and that he was left alone and left hungry	December: his birthday, Christmas May 2015: removal from family; first move into foster home for a night; went to live with great aunt July 2015: moves to foster home no. 2 October 2016: moves to foster home no. 3 (Linda)

History of family moves (e.g. moves in and out of foster care; kinship care; number of moves, attempted reunification; dates of moves between families)

1. Family home to emergency foster parent no. 1, May 2015
2. Foster parent no. 1 to great aunt, May 2015
3. Great aunt to foster parent no. 2, July 2015
4. Foster parent no. 2 to foster parent no. 3 (Linda), October 2016

Symptoms of trauma (e.g. generalized anxiety, self-harm, aggression and violence; demand avoidant; stealing, lying, nonsense chatter, attention needing; sexualized behaviours)

Aggression and violence; some sexualized language (mild); incidents of sexualized behaviour. Inability to manage school with overwhelmed violence and aggression. Showing signs of jealousy of Linda's grandchild
Josh has a great deal of superficial charm and quickly 'befriends' people

Current issues

October 2016: Josh has had multiple moves between families. Josh is presenting with a developmental age of two emotionally. Josh is developing strong feelings for Linda. This has caused a fragile attachment. Josh is having extremely violent episodes and targeting Linda. When he calms down he seeks comfort and proximity. Josh has suffered significant domestic and possible sexual abuse in the past and over a period of time. Josh has also been swearing – 'Fuck off, you bitch!' – calling Linda a 'bitch' and a 'bad mum'. He also refers to his or others' genitals a lot as 'nuts'. This behaviour is showing us trauma that he has witnessed

Event
15 November 2016: Josh and Linda were feeding the ducks and had some stale bread. Josh did not want to share. He called Linda names. His behaviour escalated, leading to him making demands for lunch and beginning to hurt Linda. He continued to escalate, punching Linda's face, shouting 'Fuck off, you bitch', also shouting that Linda should be nice to him as he had a bad time when he was little – punching and headbutting. A man who was in the area intervened, asking if everything was okay. Josh calmed down sufficiently to allow Linda to get him home. Unfortunately Josh dysregulated when he got home, and broke Linda's grandson's little chair. He carried on punching, kicking and headbutting. Linda supported Josh to go upstairs, but he headbutted and kicked her. Josh then began to calm. He stated he did not want to be angry any more and was fine. Josh later reveals that he sometimes wants to die, and discloses that his father tried to suffocate him with a blanket after Josh tried to get between his mum and dad during an argument. He also disclosed that a younger sibling was there too

Links to history
Josh was subjected to domestic violence as well as witnessing it. His language and actions are likely to replicate those that he observed, even as a very small child
He also felt he had to protect his mother from his father, and this resulted in a life-threatening situation for him. His mother was unable to protect him from his father

Strategies

The significance of this disclosure cannot be underestimated – it explains a great deal about Josh and his fears. He may believe that Linda will not be able to keep him safe and help him to survive – she is a single woman, and women have been unable to keep him safe before. Furthermore he has seen that you exert power over women, attacking them when they annoy you. This has given him a very clear precedent to follow. For his new family to maintain stability we need to support Linda to be able to find ways to reduce Josh's anxiety. In addition we can see that Josh is in despair at times – he says he wants to die. This indicates his state of mental health and also his poor internal working model – he feels worthless. He must be an awful child if his own father wanted to kill him.

This is very early on in the relationship Josh and Linda are building. When the bonding process is first happening, we call this a 'fragile' attachment. We call it 'fragile' because when the child is first beginning to feel attached to an adult, it can make them feel very vulnerable and scared. This fear can stress them to the extent that they have a full stress response. It results in 'push-me-pull-you' behaviour where the child alternately approaches and rejects the parent. He wants to be kind to Linda's grandson, but then his fears drive him away. Linda's grandson Tom is also a direct rival for Linda's attention, just as Josh is beginning to open up to her.

Josh is also scared when people arrive at the house, probably due to previous experiences of being moved on.

Strategies

Now that we have a significant amount of information, we can start to use informed strategies to help Josh and stabilize the family.

Child's name: Josh Williams   **Date of birth:** 14 December 2012

History/chronology	In utero/birth (e.g. domestic violence, drug/alcohol addiction; mental health, illness, birth trauma, premature, maternal illness, abandoned)	Antenatal (e.g. abuse, domestic violence, drug/alcohol addiction, family known to social services; unavailable mother – mental health, addictions, hospitalizations)	Known significant events/dates (e.g. hospitalizations, bereavement, date of removal from family, separation from siblings)
November 2013: family came to notice of children's services 2014: Child Protection Plan 2015: Pre-Proceedings Meeting May 2015: emergency foster care for one night after being left home alone May 2015: went to live with maternal great aunt; concerns due to her health issues July 2015: Interim Care Order granted; moves into foster family no. 1 October 2016: moves into Linda's care	Exposure to domestic violence – likelihood of high circulating cortisol	Domestic violence – this may mean increased circulating cortisol Josh has disclosed that his father touched him and that he was left alone and left hungry	December: his birthday, Christmas May 2015: removal from family; first move into foster home for a night; went to live with great aunt July 2015: moves to foster home no. 2 October 2016: moves to foster home no. 3 (Linda)

History of family moves (e.g. moves in and out of foster care; kinship care; number of moves, attempted reunification; dates of moves between families)

1. Family home to emergency foster parent no. 1, May 2015
2. Foster parent no. 1 to great aunt, May 2015
3. Great aunt to foster parent no. 2, July 2015
4. Foster parent no. 2 to foster parent no. 3 (Linda), October 2016

Symptoms of trauma (e.g. generalized anxiety, self-harm, aggression and violence; demand avoidant; stealing, lying, nonsense chatter, attention needing; sexualized behaviours)

Aggression and violence; some sexualized language (mild); incidents of sexualized behaviour. Inability to manage school with overwhelmed violence and aggression. Showing signs of jealousy of Linda's grandchild
Josh has a great deal of superficial charm and quickly 'befriends' people

Current issues

October 2016: Josh has had multiple moves between families. Josh is presenting with a developmental age of two emotionally. Josh is developing strong feelings for Linda. This has caused a fragile attachment. Josh is having extremely violent episodes and targeting Linda. When he calms down he seeks comfort and proximity. Josh has suffered significant domestic and possible sexual abuse in the past and over a period of time. Josh has also been swearing – 'Fuck off, you bitch!' – calling Linda a 'bitch' and a 'bad mum'. He also refers to his or others' genitals a lot as 'nuts'. This behaviour is showing us trauma that he has witnessed

Event

15 November 2016: Josh and Linda were feeding the ducks and had some stale bread. Josh did not want to share. He called Linda names. His behaviour escalated, leading to him making demands for lunch and beginning to hurt Linda. He continued to escalate, punching Linda's face, shouting 'Fuck off, you bitch', also shouting that Linda should be nice to him as he had a bad time when he was little – punching and headbutting. A man who was in the area intervened, asking if everything was okay. Josh calmed down sufficiently to allow Linda to get him home. Unfortunately Josh dysregulated when he got home, and broke Linda's grandson's little chair. He carried on punching, kicking and headbutting. Linda supported Josh to go upstairs, but he headbutted and kicked her. Josh then began to calm. He stated he did not want to be angry any more and was fine. Josh later reveals that he sometimes wants to die, and discloses that his father tried to suffocate him with a blanket after Josh tried to get between his mum and dad during an argument. He also disclosed that a younger sibling was there too

Links to history

Josh was subjected to domestic violence as well as witnessing it. His language and actions are likely to replicate those that he observed even as a very small child

He also felt he had to protect his mother from his father, and this resulted in a life-threatening situation for him. His mother was unable to protect him from his father

Strategies

The supporting team have been enabling Linda to have protected time with her grandson Tom. The attachment therapist and the empathic listener have worked together to give Linda narratives to use with Josh

A visual timetable has been devised so that Josh knows where he is going, when and with whom, which also clearly shows he always goes back to Linda

Josh says that he is 'bad' and that he is going to be like his dad. This is his fearfulness coming out, that the only way he has to be powerful is to be like his dad. His dad was terrifying for him. Talking to him about his fears and his fearful behaviours, it is useful to say, 'I think I see what is happening. When you are scared you remember your dad. He used to hit your mum and he hurt you. You felt so scared. I am so sorry that happened to you. You should never have been hurt like that. Remember that we are all/I am keeping you safe.' Or: 'When you are scared I think it makes you think you need to fight. You saw your dad hit your mum a lot and he was very scary! I am so sorry that happened to you. Remember, in this house we do not fight, and we are safe.' If he has been showing his conflict around Linda's grandson, remind him that we know he wants to be like a lovely big brother to Tom. We are all going to help him to practise being safe in a family. When he does kind things like getting toys out we can let him know that we can see how much he wants to be kind to Tom – but let's set him up to succeed by having greatly reduced interactions

We can talk to him about how difficult it is to belong: 'I know it is hard to be in a family because families have been so scary, and I know you are trying really hard. Remember you are safe now.' We need to remember that he witnessed violence for three years before he was removed, which was male on female, and that his father tried to kill him for trying to protect his mum. Families *are* terrifying

NEXT STEPS

We have found these strategies effective over time in helping to maintain the stability of families like Josh's.

Of course, any child like Josh will experience further challenges down the road, and his Trauma Tracker stops at a particular moment in time, purely for the purposes of serving as an example of a Trauma Tracker in this book.

But this is not where we want to stop.

Strategies are fine and can clearly offer support during challenging times, but we want to enable *lifelong* changes to be made. In order to start to try and heal the child, the next step is to consider what developmental gaps they may have, and to begin to address these alongside the narratives and support shown above.

This is long-term work that is intended to shift the perception of the child and enable them to have a revised internal working model when applied consistently, predictably and reliably.

Next we will look at Josh's unmet needs using another tool, developed by Sarah Dillon, called the Developmental Foundation Planner.

After this, we will describe how the 'Behaviour – Assessment of Impact and Resolution Tool' (BAIRT) developed by Sarah Naish can be used to help when, after a long period of relative calm, Linda becomes perplexed as Josh suddenly starts to revert to his previous aggressive behaviours.

This part has been about preparation and early days. Although a Trauma Tracker can be undertaken at any time, the ideal time to do this is prior to moving in with the family.

Top tips for welcoming a child into your home are:

- Be low key – it is stressful enough to change your home without having to manage lots of introduction and excitement.
- Take time as a family to get to know each other.
- Do not overwhelm the child with rules – keep everything simple.
- Help the child unpack at their pace. Ask them about the significance of personal objects.
- Help the child to feel welcome by using their sheets or bedding, or by cooking their favourite meal.
- Connect by spending time with them, playing alongside them, talking to them.
- Have a visual timetable ready and get a routine and structure in place from the outset.

More information about transitions can be found in Naish (2018, Part 1, Chapter 1; also on pp.164, 249, 309).

REMEMBER SELF-CARE

Readers will, I hope, be very aware that, even when things are going well, the going can still be tough and feel relentless for the parent – and this is why when we are working with families one of the things we absolutely emphasize is the need for self-care. Self-care means taking time for you, and can be any or all of the following:

- Arranging a short break to rest, recuperate and meet up with friends and family.
- Walking, swimming or other exercise.
- Yoga, meditation, mindfulness training, wellbeing and relaxation groups.
- Attending a support group.
- Phoning a friend.
- Speaking to the empathic listener.
- Taking 5 minutes to put your feet up with a cup of tea.
- Reading.
- Watching junk TV.
- Spending time with your partner or a close friend – maybe when the children are at school.
- Joining a supportive organization, such as the National Association of Therapeutic Parents.[3]

We will now move on to the Developmental Foundation Planner, and see how this was used to establish and meet Josh's unmet needs.

---

3   www.naotp.com

Part Two

Building the Cornerstones: The Developmental Foundation Planner

SARAH DILLON

The Developmental Foundation Planner is a tool that essentially takes the form of a series of tables to be completed and has been devised for supporting professionals to help parents meet the unmet developmental needs of children from trauma.

Many parents and supporting professionals who are caring for children with a history of trauma and neglect feel that they don't know where to begin. This tool establishes what each individual child's needs are and how to address them.

The first part of this Planner is the background to using the tool. Reading this is vital as it gives all the information necessary to complete the tool, although some readers may find it useful to look at the completed tool example for Josh prior to reading the Planner.

As with all the tools that feature in this resource, the Developmental Foundation Planner is intended to be used by readers already familiar with the knowledge contained in *The A–Z* (Naish 2018), which gives the correct therapeutic parenting strategies and solutions when caring for children from trauma.

The term 'parent' is used to describe anyone looking after such children in their own homes. Where I have mentioned 'caregiver', this is used to include staff who work in residential settings, teachers or others in caring roles.

THE WHY, WHAT AND HOW OF CHILDREN'S BEHAVIOUR

Throughout my work with families, I always begin with 'why' a child behaves in the way they do because a thorough understanding of this is vital if we are to deliver effective re-parenting. Many parents and supporting professionals focus on a child's behaviours and are seeking to understand 'how' to manage these behaviours. This can be extremely frustrating for all involved as many standard behavioural strategies actually exacerbate the problem! So a thorough understanding of 'why' will ensure we use the correct 'how'.

Further to this, the strategies indicated by this tool will not be successful without the essential empathy and nurture to support both the adults and the child, and these come most easily with understanding. This is why I use the following formula when helping parents to understand their child's behaviour and to meet their unmet needs:

Why: Why is the child behaving this way?

What: What, exactly, are they doing, and which of their behaviours are the result of the why?

How: How do we help the child and reduce the behaviours?

The Developmental Foundation Planner tool follows this 'why – what – how' formula, and it is vital for everyone involved to remember that the 'why' ultimately informs the 'how'.

UNDERSTANDING THE IMPACT OF UNMET DEVELOPMENTAL NEEDS

I am well known for my saying 'An unmet need remains unmet until it's met'.

This raises three questions:

1. What are those needs?
2. How do we establish which of them are unmet in an individual child?
3. How do we meet those needs?

Children who have experienced trauma and neglect have many unmet developmental needs, and meeting those needs is an essential part of therapeutic parenting.

I often use the analogy of building a house for parenting a child: it is essential that we lay cornerstones and have firm foundations. However, children who have been traumatized and neglected between the ages of zero and four years including prenatally have not adequately experienced the developmental foundation on which to build.

Further to this, many such children have experienced trauma that the vast majority of adults have, thankfully, never been exposed to.

These experiences affect the developmental age of the child, so before working on the cornerstones we need to recognize that by parenting them at their chronological age we are not addressing the developmental gaps that arise from developmental trauma.

Although the child may be eight years old 'chronologically', that is, they have been alive for eight years, we cannot assume that they have fully engaged in normal healthy living for that period. Indeed, for much of their history they have been in a state of survival, and this is why it is necessary to be constantly aware of this when parenting them.

In *The A–Z*, Sarah Naish (2018, p.262) emphasizes developmental gaps:

Look at the child's emotional age. If the behaviour is telling you that there are big developmental gaps where the child cannot meet the milestones (for example, of being unsupervised, playing alone) then lower your expectations accordingly. If you gauge the child at six months of age, go back to that stage.

Sadly, many supporting professionals have not had the necessary training around understanding trauma and are not fully aware of these developmental gaps. This means that when children come into care or are placed with adoptive families, parents are told to parent their children at their biological age. This sets the child and parent up to fail, particularly when they reach adolescence.

We are all aware of how many family breakdowns and unplanned endings occur for teens in care. This is because we are trying to put a roof on their house without those firm foundations, and inevitably the whole thing collapses! As a result, as mentioned by Sarah in the 'Introduction', many supporting professionals find themselves working in a way that is *reactive* as opposed to *proactive*.

Many young people who may have appeared 'settled' in their families are now bounced around the system. Adoptive and foster parents are often 'blamed' because professionals not trained in this area cannot understand why the child has unravelled.

Further to this, we also need to consider birth children who have not experienced neglect but who may have experienced trauma that has impeded their emotional development. This could be for a number of reasons. The following list, although not exhaustive, gives some common ones:

- Trauma experienced in the womb due to ill health of the mother or to high cortisol levels due to stress, grief, pregnancy complications or living in unsafe or unsettled environments whilst pregnant.
- Difficult and traumatic birth.
- Postnatal depression.
- Medical interventions.
- Relationship breakdowns.
- Domestic abuse.
- Parental alienation.
- Anxious parenting due to parents recovering from or managing their own historical trauma.
- Loss or lack of support network.
- Hospitalization of either parent or child.
- Contact issues if parents have separated.

Such traumatic experiences in early childhood can have far-reaching or even lifelong consequences regarding emotional development if not addressed.

It should be noted that some children are more resilient than others, particularly if they are securely attached, but an awareness of the impact of such experiences can be very helpful if we are struggling to understand a child's behaviour or are unsuccessful in obtaining a firm diagnosis for them. I often describe this as the 'tentacles of trauma' reaching out from early childhood and affecting the child as they grow up.

This is explained well in the 'Introduction' in *The A–Z*:

> Therapeutic parenting is also used for biological parents, particularly where there may have been pre-birth trauma, separation, illness or any other factor affecting the child's functioning and understanding of the world, or affecting their attachment. Many biological parents find therapeutic parenting styles useful to use with children who are

on the autism spectrum or have high cortisol levels and/or attention deficit hyperactivity disorder (ADHD). (Naish 2018, p.13)

There is also an overview of Developmental Trauma Disorder and other diagnoses in Chapter 2 (Naish 2018, pp.29–31).

We also need to consider the sensory needs of children with developmental trauma. My experience has been that most children who have experienced early-life trauma will have some sensory difficulties, typically with sounds or sudden noise, certain lighting, a need to chew things or finding certain skin sensations (such as labels in clothes) intolerable, and these can lead to extreme dysregulation in such children. Sarah discusses this further in Chapter 1 of *The A–Z* (Naish 2018, pp.26–27).

THE FOUR CORNERSTONES OF THERAPEUTIC PARENTING

After working with many hundreds of parents I have been able to identify four fundamental areas of unmet developmental needs, which I call the 'cornerstones' of therapeutic parenting. They are:

1. Establishing the parent as the unassailable safe base.
2. Developing object permanence.
3. Regular relationship repairs.
4. Linking cause and effect.

In Chapter 3 of *The A–Z*, Sarah expands on the importance of boundaries and structure:

Therapeutic parenting is founded primarily on boundaries and structure. It is not possible to use the more effective strands to therapeutic parenting without this essential foundation. Our children often come from a place where they were lacking the structure of routine, boundaries and safety, so the first way we can help them to feel safe enough to learn and grow is by making their lives predictable. (Naish 2018, p.32)

In considering the four cornerstones we will see how boundaries and structure help to get the cornerstones firmly in place so that we can begin to meet the unmet needs.

However, identifying which needs are unmet is not straightforward, not least because these needs are most commonly communicated via the child's behaviours and are rarely expressed verbally.

Once we support a parent to focus on each cornerstone, we begin to meet those unmet developmental needs and indeed begin to lay a firm developmental foundation on which the child can build.

As with building a house, all four cornerstones are essential. When applying these to the developmental needs of the child we must always begin with the first cornerstone, establishing an adult as their unassailable safe base (a concept introduced on p.33 of *The A–Z*). The other three cornerstones can only be laid when the first is firmly in place, and none of them work in isolation.

The Developmental Foundation Planner tool helps us to identify which cornerstone or stones need strengthening in any particular child, and I believe it is important that we use this tool to support parents to begin to meet the unmet developmental needs of all children who have experienced trauma and neglect.

Throughout my work I meet many children and young people who exhibit behaviours more closely associated with that of a toddler but, because they are biologically older, society expects them to behave accordingly. Sarah puts this succinctly in the 'Introduction' of *The A–Z*:

> We always try to think about our children's emotional age, and not their chronological age, as, to be honest, their chronological age is not very relevant. (Naish 2018, p.14)

Indeed, we see many children leaving care who are still emotionally and developmentally much younger than their chronological age.

Any child who has experienced trauma and neglect in the first few years of life will have developed a negative internal working model. This means that they do not feel safe. They believe they are intrinsically bad and, due to infant egocentricity, they are convinced that, if they have had any influence on the world, it is a negative one. Some feel that they have had no impact whatsoever on the world around them.

Chapter 1 of *The A–Z* explains the child's internal working model:

> The child gets their sense of self from the actions of the people around them. If they are ignored or abused, their sense of self is one of worthlessness and 'badness'. Guilt can be described as 'I did something bad'. Shame is more like 'I am bad' [Brown 2012]. This feeling of 'badness' is internalized, so the child's internal working model might be, 'I am bad, I am unimportant, I am unlovable.' It is not a decision they have made, it is the way their brain has been wired. (Naish 2018, p.25)

Further to this, they do not believe that adults will keep them safe or that they are consistent, predictable and reliable, and therefore the child will not invest in a trusting relationship with their primary caregiver. It is, however, this relationship that is pivotal to the development of the child, and so, when we concentrate our focus on the four cornerstones, we will enable the child to begin to invest in a trusting relationship with their parent.

After exploring each cornerstone we will be able to see that, in addressing them, we are also meeting many other developmental needs along the way. As we begin to meet these needs we will initially see some developmental regression, and we may need to help parents to give support with a number of the following issues:

- Washing and dressing.
- Toilet training.
- Wanting to use a bottle or soother.
- Playing with toys according to their developmental or emotional age.
- Preferring the company of much younger children.
- Needing to sleep with or beside a parent.
- Bedroom may need to be simplified with regards to belongings, toys, etc.
- Need for rocking and cradling.
- Speaking in a 'baby' voice or babbling.

- Crawling.
- Being fed.

We need not be concerned by these behaviours. They are a sign that the child is feeling safe enough to 'show' their caregivers what they have not had. Throughout my work, I have found that in order for a child to progress, they first need to regress. The associated behaviours are often described by those caring for such children as 'immaturity' (see Naish 2018, pp.179–182).

Let's consider how unmet early-life needs are communicated via behaviours in older children.

Our children have complex behaviours that arise from many underlying factors. In Chapter 1 of *The A–Z*, Sarah states:

> Many of the behaviours we see in our children are fear-based responses, but they may not appear to us in that way. Indeed, our child may present as rude, defiant and attention-seeking… [If we] start from the basis that a child who has suffered some kind of trauma in their early life often feels out of control and experiences the world very differently, some of their behaviours start to make sense. (Naish 2018, p.19)

She describes fear-based behaviours under the following headings (Naish 2018, pp.20–24):

- Fear.
- Unable to re-attune.
- Blocked trust.
- Impulsivity.
- Lack of cause-and-effect thinking.
- Control and power issues.
- Lack of empathy.
- Lack of remorse.
- Hypervigilance.
- Sadness, grief and loss.
- Fear of invisibility.
- Anger.

Consequently, children from trauma can:

- Be superficially engaging and charming.
- Lack eye contact on adult terms.
- Be indiscriminately affectionate with strangers or not affectionate at all.
- Be destructive of self, others and material things.
- Be cruel to animals.
- Steal or take things.
- Self-harm.
- Have outbursts of aggression or tantrums.
- Struggle with transitions.

- Abscond.
- Lie.
- Lack impulse control.
- Frequently be hyperactive.
- Have learning delays.
- Lack development of cause-and-effect thinking.
- Lack conscience, empathy and compassion.
- Have abnormal eating patterns.
- Have poor peer relationships.
- Engage in incessant chatter or nonsense questions.
- Follow people around.
- Be rude, defiant and controlling.
- Have issues around toileting.
- Have sleep issues.

Caring for a child with such behaviour is exhausting, and sadly, children who display many of these behaviours often move between numerous foster homes or have to leave their adoptive families and go back into care. Worse, a number of them are eventually moved to a residential setting without a consistent and ever-present caregiver, which further impacts independent living as there is no parental safe base to return to.

Many children who leave care without a safe parental base to return to experience serious mental health problems, homelessness and addictions, and may well have their own children taken into care.

We need to look at these behaviours through a different lens. If we read back over the list we can easily see that such behaviours could be attributed to any toddler, and we would say they are absolutely developmentally normal. Of course, the behaviours would be far less intense and it is much easier to manage these behaviours in a small child than it is in an older child or well-developed teen.

This is why standard age-dependent parenting strategies do not work for children who have experienced early-life trauma and neglect (see Chapter 6 in Naish 2018, pp.59–67).

Chapter 5 of *The A–Z* reinforces the need to set our expectations so that they are consistent with the child's capabilities and emotional age:

> If we expect the child to be able to function emotionally and developmentally at their chronological age, we are most likely setting everyone up to fail, including ourselves. When setting boundaries, set them for the emotional age. (Naish 2018, p.52)

EFFECTIVE USE OF THE DEVELOPMENTAL FOUNDATION PLANNER

In order to use the tool effectively, we begin by looking at each cornerstone. Understanding how these fundamental unmet needs are communicated via specific behaviours enables us to identify developmental gaps in an individual child.

Historical chronology helps to identify unmet developmental needs, particularly where there has been significant neglect. Current presenting behaviours can be better understood through the lens of this chronology. The Trauma Tracker in Part One of this book enables us to use this lens effectively.

Where this historical information is either limited or unavailable, the gaps can still be deduced from behaviour, and the example tool at the end shows this in practice.

Once we have identified the specific cornerstones in need of strengthening, we can introduce the correct approach and strategies.

Each cornerstone is laid out in the following order:

- Cornerstone explained.
- Associated presenting behaviours.
- Therapeutic parenting approach and strategies.

CORNERSTONE 1: ESTABLISHING THE PARENT AS THE UNASSAILABLE SAFE BASE

Cornerstone explained

A child without an adult as an unassailable safe base is alone in a scary and hostile world, adrift, and unable to rely on having any of their needs met.

The first thing we need to focus on when establishing a parent as an unassailable safe base is 'claiming' the child. For most children and parents, claiming starts in the womb. We don't just give birth and start loving the baby only when it's born. In most cases, our love for a baby begins early on in the pregnancy.

A woman will claim her baby whilst she is pregnant, talking and singing to the baby in the womb, knowing that they can hear and will come to recognize the parent's voice. Often both parents will gently touch and rub the pregnant belly or massage it, respond to the baby's kicks, play music to the baby. They will spend time reflecting, thinking about the baby, and will probably have an ultrasound and see the baby moving about the womb. During such times the baby's developing brain in utero is flooded with hormones, such as oxytocin, which have a positive effect on bonding, and the baby is conditioned to feel safe. When they are born they feel safe enough to enter into a positive attachment cycle with their caregiver.

What if your child did not experience this? Perhaps their birth parent was very anxious during pregnancy and the baby's brain was flooded with stress hormones such as cortisol. This means that the baby is wired for danger when they are born. They could be hyper-aroused (on high alert) or hypo-aroused (under-responsive). Either way, there will be a rupture in the developing attachment the child forms with the primary caregiver. This can be a particular problem for adoptive parents, who may assume that because their child was removed at birth they will have no lasting difficulties.

However, the child needs to survive, and they will develop maladaptive ways, also known as insecure attachment patterns, in order to get their needs met. Much of the training we are currently able to access focuses on the intersubjective relationship between a child and their parent after the child is born. It is necessary for the baby to enter into this attuned relationship in which the parent will interpret the behaviour of the baby, identify and meet their needs, and become their regulatory figure.

If a child has not been adequately claimed and has not entered into a reliable and intersubjective relationship, they will be stuck using behaviour to communicate their unmet developmental needs and the trauma they have experienced in the same way that any baby uses behaviour to communicate what they need and how they feel.

Further to this, they will struggle to identify their own needs and feelings, including their need to be in control to feel safe. Many of them cannot ask an adult for help due to the lack of a reciprocal relationship as babies. This culminates in fear-based behaviours and the child can become extremely controlling and hypervigilant.

Sarah (Naish 2018, p.21) expresses it thus:

> It's also very disconcerting to realize that, often, what our children are most scared of are adults. This is upsetting for parents and something they may not have considered. If your child appears to be rejecting everything, is unable to ask for help and follows you around, seemingly ever watchful, consider that *you may be the source of fear as well as comfort*. (emphasis added)

When thinking about this we need to understand that, although much attention needs to be paid to the development of the intersubjective relationship between parent and child, we can only really begin to do this once we have found a way of claiming the child. Claiming a child will significantly reduce their fear-based responses as they begin to feel safe and develop trust that a parent will meet their needs.

Sadly, many foster parents in particular are still taught not to get too close to the child in case they have to move, but then they are given training that encourages them to attach to the child. This leaves foster parents in a very difficult situation as they are unsure how close they are allowed to get to a child, particularly as they are not the legal parent.

Unfortunately, there are still some supporting professionals who advise foster parents not to touch the child. Not only is this wrong, but it is also extremely rejecting and emotionally damaging for the child. Can you imagine *never* being hugged or touched?

I am well aware of the need for safeguarding and each child is different but, as a profession, we have become so risk-averse that many children are being deprived of the most basic need for human connection!

We should not drown a traumatized child in affection and we most definitely need to be aware of historical abuse and allegations etc., but this must *not* stop us from seeking ways to comfort them and offer affection. For some children, this might only be a gentle touch on the shoulder rather than a warm embrace, but it is still necessary nonetheless.

I believe that even if a child is only placed with a foster parent for a short time, they still need the experience of being 'claimed'. A parent can easily communicate their joy at having the child with them, even if only for a day. Claiming is vital when establishing a parent as the child's safe base because the child needs to believe they are important to their parent.

When delivering training I'll often focus on a process called 'belong, believe, behave'. I am convinced that if we can help a child to belong, eventually they will believe that the relationship with the parent is worth investing in and, as a result of that, we see a reduction in behaviours.

Belong: The child feels secure and wanted

Believe: The child feels safe and able to 'risk' entering into a relationship with the adult

Behave: The child's behaviours reduce as their fear diminishes; they are regulated by the adult

For all children who have experienced trauma and neglect, behaviour is their loudest voice. For some of our children, behaviour is their only voice. Once we begin to meet their unmet developmental needs, there is a reduction in the communication of those needs by the behaviours.

In order for a child to access an adult as an unassailable safe base they first need to believe that they are wanted by the adult.

One of the problems that we face when children come into care, particularly into foster homes, is that we need to become everything that the child needs. Although this may be true, we also need to consider that children who have experienced trauma and neglect do not feel that adults can meet their needs, and so they don't believe that they require adults in the same way that a neurotypical child would. Sarah describes this as 'blocked trust':

> If the child has not learned that the parent or carer is reliable and trustworthy then they are unable to rely on them to meet even their basic needs. Our children are often mistrustful of our intentions and find it difficult to interpret our actions, even to read facial expressions. (Naish 2018, p.21)

Let us now think about the first few months of a baby's life. When a baby is born, the parents will spend much time adoring and delighting in the child. There will be a period of bonding when there is a nurture bubble created around the parents and the child. During this time the parents will seek to establish a strong routine for the baby. They will spend much time holding and stroking the baby, getting up in the night, talking and singing to the baby, enabling the baby to access the parents for comfort and co-regulation.

It is this experience that underpins the child's developing attachment to the parent. The child feels that they are having a positive impact on their world. The child feels claimed and needed by the parent. This, in turn, helps to promote the development of the positive internal working model in such a baby, thus developing self-esteem, self-worth, warmth and affection.

Children who have been exposed to trauma and neglect may never have experienced such claiming and so do not perceive the adult as their safe base; in turn, they convince themselves that they do not need the adult. Furthermore, they do not believe that they are having a positive impact on the world. Sadly, their main purpose for staying in a relationship with the adult is to stay alive, to make sure their needs, even the ones only subconsciously felt, are met, and to keep them safe.

We therefore need to find ways to help a child from trauma and neglect to feel that their very existence has brought positivity to their parents' lives. This might be by helping the child to realize that if they were not with them, their family would not function effectively.

Associated presenting behaviours

Which specific behaviours may we see arising from not having a sense of the parent as an unassailable safe base? Most, but not all, such children will exhibit behaviours from one or other of the following lists. Note that some behaviours occur in both lists.

AVOIDING ADULTS

- Avoiding adults to keep safe.
- Not asking for help.
- Hiding in their bedroom.
- Saying that everything is fine when it's not.
- Not trusting adults to meet their needs.
- Believing that it is only a matter of time before they are moved on.
- Rejecting adults.
- Unable to access adults for comfort and co-regulation.
- Innate need to be in control.
- Lack of sense of belonging.
- Failing to follow instructions from an adult whilst pretending to do so.
- Overly compliant.
- Disingenuous and inauthentic (masking).
- Secretive.
- Cannot self-regulate.
- Withdrawn and insular.

BEFRIENDING ADULTS

- Befriending adults to keep safe.
- Fake smiling.
- Anxious and clingy.
- Not trusting adults to meet their needs.
- Believing that it is only a matter of time before they are moved on.
- Unable to genuinely access adults for comfort and co-regulation.
- Innate need to be in control.
- People-pleasing.
- Lack of sense of belonging.
- Failing to follow instructions from an adult.
- Overly compliant.
- Disingenuous and inauthentic (masking).
- Cannot self-regulate.
- Pretending to share the adult's interests.

In addition to the above, some children are so terrified of adults, due to extreme trauma, that they become highly aggressive, destructive and violent. These children will do almost anything to avoid accessing an adult as their safe base.

I often use the following analogy:

If you are scared of something, really scared, what do you do? Say you have a phobia of spiders and one suddenly appears. What happens? You might freeze and feel panicky. You may try and run away, or even kill it. You can't think straight. You might keep a very close eye on that spider so you know where it is at all times. Well, I felt that way about adults. Adults were the source of my trauma and phobia, and every time I was moved I had a new spider to get used to.

Therapeutic parenting approach and strategies

What strategies might we use in order to establish a parent as the child's safe base?

'CLAIMING' VOCABULARY

The first thing is to encourage a parent to begin using a 'claiming' vocabulary. It is extremely powerful to preface the child's name with 'my' or 'our', but with due regard to whether or not the child is receptive to being claimed at this particular moment. Parents must not let their fear of claiming a child, or their response to such an attempt, deter them from doing so, although they may need to choose their moments.

STAYING CLOSE OR PARENTAL PRESENCE

When considering the fact that children from trauma may not have effectively experienced co-regulation via an attuned and available caregiver, they have significant problems around self-regulation. This means they struggle to calm down on their own.

Imagine a radiator and its necessary thermostat. Unfortunately, if the thermostat is faulty or absent, the radiator will not be able to regulate its heat. In the same way, a child with Developmental Trauma Disorder cannot self-regulate. The parent needs to become their thermostat, which also means that they need to be both present and regulated themselves in order to regulate the child. When establishing a parent as the unassailable safe base, it is vitally important that they seek ways to calm themselves first in order to help the child to do the same.

CHILD'S OWN PLACES AND THINGS

Beyond vocabulary, allocating a specific chair to the child in the living room, having their own seat at the table, perhaps their own crockery and cutlery, will help the child to feel they have a place in the family (see Naish 2018, pp.125–126).

GIVING THE CHILD A TASK

Asking the child to help the parent with something and thanking them afterwards, letting them know that they have a job in the home that only they can do, will help them to feel that they can have a positive impact in their new family and that they are needed, wanted and have a purpose.

When I was in care, my foster mum gave me the task of cleaning the bathroom. It made me feel that I had an important role in the family. When I announced one day that I was leaving, she said, 'Oh my goodness, what would we do without you? Who's going to clean the bathroom?' I remember feeling needed and decided to stay. To this day, my bathroom is the cleanest room in the house!

ROUTINE

Establish a strong routine for the child. This is the first of the foundations for therapeutic parenting (Naish 2018, Chapter 3), and is essential in establishing the parent as the safe and unassailable base.

Routines give children a sense of security and help them to develop a belief that life can be predictable. Routines promote that sense of belonging in the family, remind the child that their needs will be met – dinner time, play time, bath time, story time and bed time. Repetition is necessary to encourage new synaptic development in the brain; this 'rewiring' of the brain is essential for successful outcomes for children who have experienced trauma and neglect.

In the 'Introduction' in *The A–Z* Sarah underlines the importance of routine:

> Therapeutic parents live a life that is well structured with strict routines and boundaries. There are no surprises or spontaneous outings and there is no room for doubt. This can be dull at times and frustrating for everyone. The strict routines may be misinterpreted as inflexibility by extended family or supporting professionals. Therapeutic parents often long for spontaneity and a change to routine, but have learned, to their cost, that there is always a price to pay for these deviations! (Naish 2018, p.14)

BOUNDARIES

Strong and firm boundaries underpin therapeutic parenting. Children feel safe when a consistent and reliable adult is in charge. Boundary setting creates scaffolding around a child's emotional development. If we consider children aged two to seven, their world is usually full of wonder, often described as 'magical thinking'. This means they are not equipped to make big decisions. The therapeutic parent is at the 'helm of the ship' at all times.

When speaking at conferences or delivering training, I am often asked about my experience of being in care. I use the analogy of walking along the edge of a cliff wearing a blindfold. Thankfully, the wonderful foster mum with whom I finally settled was like a wall at the side of the cliff, which helped me to feel very safe even though I rebelled against it. Once she had implemented a boundary, she didn't move it. I firmly believe that this enabled me to begin to rely on her as my unassailable safe base. Sometimes I described her as my 'Mount Kilimanjaro'. She could not be moved!

VISUAL TIMETABLES

Visual timetables really help parents to keep on track with the child throughout the day. If a child has had many moves within the care system, they are conditioned to believe it is only a matter of time before they are moved again. However, a visual timetable can reassure a child that they will still be with their family today, tomorrow and even next week. See the Trauma Tracker in Part One to further understand how fear of removal is also linked to intrinsically held memory of times a child has been moved in the past.

I have found that many traumatized children struggle with verbal information and respond far better to visual reminders. They need to 'see' what is happening next, and not just hear. Their anxiety can be greatly reduced as the visual timetable is a comforting reminder of predictability and can always be referred to. We need to remember that many of our children are hypervigilant and are always alert for the next bad thing to happen. Visual timetables help to alleviate this fear.

Children who have experienced developmental trauma have problems with memory and organization. The therapeutic parent has to do much of their remembering and organizing for them, and the visual timetable is an essential tool. Sarah emphasizes this in *The A–Z* (Naish 2018, p.203).

These strategies are dependent upon a parent establishing themselves as an unassailable safe base for the child and seeking ways to help the child to belong. As a result of this, the intrinsically held belief system that the child has about adults is challenged. Now we have a child who may begin to risk investing in a relationship with an adult who is able to meet their needs and keep them safe, and an adult who delights in them.

If a child struggles to engage in family rituals, it is important that the parent uses language that communicates their desire to engage with them as opposed to telling the child that they need to engage with the parent. A child will never believe that they need a parent until the adult first communicates that they are important to them and that, if they left, their lives would be diminished.

Foster children may also have continued visits with their birth family and so it is important that the caregiver helps the child to understand that they can belong in both families without feeling overwhelmed by a sense of disloyalty and shame. It is important to remember that claiming a child does not have to compromise any existing attachment to birth family.

PLAY

Children from trauma may not have learned to play. Play is often described as 'a child's work' as this is how they learn and grow as individuals. They use play to process what they think and feel and develop their imagination. Play also helps with developing dexterity and cognitive strength, and not just in humans – wildlife documentaries featuring young at play are always a delight. Children use play to work through many childhood schemas.

Schemas are usually described as patterns of repeated behaviour. Children use schemas to express developing ideas through play and exploration. The repetition of schematic play allows children to construct meaning in what they are doing, and also helps them to link cause and effect.

Remember that it is important to play with a child at their developmental age as opposed to their chronological age. We cannot expect a child from trauma to play independently. This will only happen once we have taught them how to play. We should encourage parents to use toys more suited to a toddler where possible.

EMPATHIC COMMENTARY

Empathic commentary enables us to develop a narrative around what we see a child doing and link that back to how that child may be feeling. This, in turn, helps the child to see that their primary caregiver is attuned with them, that this adult has taken time to see beyond the child's behaviours to those early-life unmet needs of being claimed (see Naish 2018, p.45).

'NAMING THE NEED'

I often call 'naming the need' 'the gift of why'. Due to a traumatized child's negative internal working model, the story they have about themselves and why they do the things they do is built on their belief that they are intrinsically bad.

Often when we ask a child why they have behaved in a certain way they will respond by saying they don't know, or will come up with any reason to avoid triggering overwhelming emotions connected to their negative internal working model.

Emotion is energy in motion, which indicates that it needs to move! This means that when a child is triggered by something, emotions flood the child's body and they can become distressed and dysregulated. I describe this rush of emotion as a trauma tornado spinning within the child. We have written about this in *The Quick Guide to Therapeutic Parenting* (Naish and Dillon 2020).

It is important that we help parents to create a narrative around what the child is doing or experiencing and link this back to their early-life unmet developmental needs and traumatic experiences. When parents use this strategy, it gives the child an alternative lens through which to view themselves and their behaviours. This, in turn, dilutes the triggered emotional response and can sometimes calm the child quite quickly.

When establishing the parent as the unassailable safe base, it is very helpful to the child to know that the parent is able to identify how current behaviours can link directly to unmet needs in early childhood. This increases the child's sense of safety as the therapeutic parent knows everything!

An example of 'naming the need' is as follows. A child does not want to engage in family activities and chooses to remain in their room most of the time. The therapeutic parent might say:

> I have noticed you're spending a lot of time in your room, not wanting to do things with us as a family. I think this is because you spent a lot of time in your bedroom when you were little and it's scary to spend time with us. I'll work hard to help you with these feelings as we miss having you with us.

A word of caution: children from trauma are fearful of intimacy, because intimacy is 'in to me see'. As they believe they are bad, they are fearful of the parent seeing their badness, and therefore they may reject the parent's insight. If this happens, the parent needs to empathize with the child, stick to the narrative, and offer to apologize later if they're wrong.

CORNERSTONE 2: DEVELOPING OBJECT PERMANENCE

Cornerstone explained

Object permanence typically starts to develop between four and seven months of age, and involves a baby's understanding that even when they can't see an object, it is still there. Before the baby understands this concept, things that leave the baby's view have ceased to exist.

Developing object permanence is a fundamental milestone. To develop object permanence we may play things like peek-a-boo and hide-and-seek etc., but in reality, the development of object permanence relies on far more than play.

When a baby has a need and a parent consistently and predictably responds to that need, the baby is conditioned to believe that even though a parent may leave their view, they still exist. When we consistently return after leaving the room to retrieve a bottle or a nappy, or reliably respond to them in the night by offering comfort and co-regulation, the baby comes to know that the parent still exists even when they can't see them. This knowledge of the adult's continued existence is why neurotypical children can generally cope with delayed gratification, for example by playing or waiting contentedly until the adult returns. I refer to this as 'parental permanence'.

This is the process by which the child further internalizes the parent as their primary attachment figure and safe base. It means that the child can access the parent for comfort which aids regulation even when they are apart.

Children who have experienced trauma and neglect have not developed object permanence sufficiently. This means that an older child who is in care can re-experience a sense of abandonment every time their primary caregiver is out of their line of sight.

Associated presenting behaviours

Which behaviours may we see arising from a lack of well-developed object permanence?

- A child may follow us everywhere.
- A child may constantly chatter and ask nonsense questions through fear of invisibility and fear of being forgotten.
- Often, these children have numerous sleep issues. They may struggle to go to sleep at night because they intrinsically believe that when the adult leaves the room they are no longer available for them, particularly if nobody consistently got up to them in the night when they were babies.
- Some of these children cannot stay asleep as they need to frequently check the availability of adults. They will keep calling the adult's name or come downstairs to make sure the adult is still there.
- A child may repeatedly say 'hello' to an adult whenever they walk back into a room after a brief absence (for example, a toilet break or to make a cuppa), as if they've been away for a significant period of time.
- We may also see problems in school because once the parent has left the child at school the child struggles to believe that the parent still exists and, indeed, that they will return to collect them at the end of the day. This is further compounded by uninformed social workers who enter into schools and either take children into care or move them to a new foster home. I have personally experienced this and can still remember watching the classroom door or running past any cars outside the school just in case a social worker 'took me away'.

Throughout *The A–Z* we see many examples of how the fear of invisibility, fear of abandonment and separation anxiety drive such behaviours:

> When a child has suffered from unreliable parenting, neglect or abuse, they may have a deep-rooted fear of being forgotten or invisible. They will certainly have felt invisible at times. If you are dependent on powerful adults to feed you and keep you safe, but you appear to be invisible, you might die. When our children are scared of being forgotten we see some of the most powerful behaviours, such as nonsense chatter, anxiety-based behaviours, following and aggressive or rude behaviours, designed to press the parent's buttons and forcibly remind them that the child is there! (Naish 2018, pp.23–24)

When we explore this further it is understandable that, due to the ruptured attachment that the child has experienced and, for some of our children, numerous ruptured attachments, they are conditioned to believe that adults are temporary figures. Adults don't stick around, and when they leave, they're gone forever.

It should be noted that children have sleep issues for many reasons (for more details see 'Sleep Issues' in Naish 2018, pp.277–283), but for the purposes of this part of the book we are focusing on this particular cornerstone, object permanence, as when we address this we are continuing to establish the parent as an unassailable safe base for the child.

Once the child begins to feel safe physically and emotionally they will begin to invest in a relationship with an adult. This cannot begin unless the child truly believes that even though they may not be able to physically see the parent, they have internalized them as their primary attachment figure and therefore know that the parent is still available, even when they are apart.

Therapeutic parenting approach and strategies

Which strategies may we use to further develop object permanence?

VISUAL TIMETABLES
Building on our use of visual timetables enables the child to physically see what is coming next, which can reduce anxiety connected to fears around adult availability.

RESPONDING TO THE NEEDS OF A CHILD
When a child has a need, especially when this is being communicated via difficult behaviours, it is important that we help parents to interpret the behaviour to figure out what the child is actually communicating and to respond to that need. When we consistently and reliably respond to and meet such needs, the child begins to internalize the adult's availability.

STAYING CLOSE
When a child is extremely dysregulated, it is important that the therapeutic parent remains in close proximity. The child needs to know that the parent is available and hasn't abandoned them when they are distressed. Sarah refers to this under 'Parental presence' in Chapter 5 of *The A–Z* (Naish 2018, p.53).

EMPATHIC COMMENTARY

Empathic commentary is one of the building blocks of therapeutic parenting. Therefore, it is a strategy or response that underpins each cornerstone. Attuned caregivers use the technique. The adult interprets and verbalizes the inner world of the child, and connects this to behaviours in the moment.

For example, we may say to a child, 'I can see that you are worried that I may not collect you from school at the end of the day. This is why you are angry when I leave you.'

Empathic commentary helps a child to understand themselves, to develop a safe narrative around their behaviours and keep the relationship with the parent intact throughout. This approach is reassuring for a child who has an underdeveloped sense of object permanence.

GETTING UP TO THE CHILD IN THE NIGHT

As a baby, if nobody got up to you in the night, you would feel that you were completely abandoned during this time.

In *The A–Z*, Sarah gives strategies for bedtime issues and explains why a child might struggle at night (Naish 2018, pp.96–97). Those applicable to this cornerstone are:

- Separation anxiety – bedtime means that there will be a prolonged separation.
- Fear of invisibility – when the child is in bed sometimes they fear they will 'disappear' or be forgotten about if they go to sleep.
- Fear of abandonment.

This is further explored in 'Sleep Issues' in *The A–Z*:

> If your child has missed out on early nurture they may well be stuck at an earlier emotional stage. Think about what your child's behaviour is saying. Is it the same as you might expect for a six-month-old? A one-year-old? It may be that the only way your child can feel completely secure all night through is to be close to their primary caregiver in the same way that a baby is with a similar routine, and then to move through the developmental stages. (Naish 2018, p.278)

A useful strategy to address this is to create a routine that includes checking on the child during the night.

What might this look like? It can be useful to use a tick-chart on the bedroom wall so that when the child is awake they have visible evidence that the parent came in to their room at certain times to see that they were safe.

The parent's language may include something like: 'I miss you at night, so I'm just going to pop in and check that you're okay.' They may say: 'When you were little, I think there may have been times when you cried for an adult to come and nobody came, which is why your brain is very worried in the night that I'm not there for you.'

Before implementing this strategy the parent needs to explain to the child what they propose doing, and why, and seek their permission. We must also take into account any historical abuse they may have experienced, particularly in the bedroom. (If the child has a social worker, we will also need to seek their permission.)

In the event of a child not wishing to engage with this strategy, the parent can post a little note under the door to let them know that they were thinking of them. The note would say something like: 'At 2 am I put my ear to your door to check that you were okay.'

We must remember that although a child may not want this intervention, the need remains unmet, and we may need to be inventive in meeting it.

During this approach the parent does not need to wake the child. They can gently stroke their brow or touch their shoulder and reassure them that they are still there and haven't forgotten them. Interestingly, the many parents who have used this strategy have told me that although the child doesn't wake, if they haven't been in the room the child will soon remind them that they did not check on them during the night.

For anybody who may have concerns about this strategy, if you find that it is triggering for a child or makes them feel unsafe in any way, then perhaps this is not the strategy for that particular child. That being said, I'm a firm believer that it can be very useful to try, and experience has shown us that there is often great success in developing object permanence when meeting this unmet need.

The purpose of this strategy is to help the child to know that even though they are not with the parent during the night, the parent hasn't forgotten them and they still exist.

SAND TIMERS AND SINGING

The use of a sand timer in helping children to actually get to sleep can be very beneficial. The therapeutic parent will usually start with about 10 or 15 minutes and ask the child to watch the sand fall through the sand timer, reassuring them that they will return as soon as the sand has emptied and they call the parent. It is important that they do return when the child calls them, at which point they will enter the room and spend a minute or two with the child, giving encouragement and reassurance that they haven't forgotten them.

This needs to be repeated for a number of weeks, but the time can be extended between leaving and returning. The child will often fall asleep quite quickly just through focusing on the sand disappearing.

If the child calls the parent before the sand has disappeared, they will need to respond empathically and remind the child that the process needs to begin again, whilst reassuring them that they understand that they're finding this difficult.

It is important to remember that people with a history of trauma are extremely hypervigilant, and this will also impact on sleep issues.

Often, when a parent has put a child to bed they will endeavour to be quiet whilst busying themselves downstairs. When helping a child develop object permanence this is not necessarily the best course of action. The saying 'the calm comes before the storm' is very apt for children from trauma who really struggle with silences. In order for them to know that you are still available for them when they are in their bedrooms it can be helpful for them to hear you moving about the house, singing and speaking.

As a former foster child I still remember listening to my foster mother singing whilst I was lying in bed at night. It was a great comfort to know that she was still there and, furthermore, not being subjected to violence.

Some of our children have been abandoned in their bedrooms for extremely long periods of time, and so it is important for them to know that we are still there, and therefore we need to make ourselves heard.

Waking in the morning can be a particularly difficult time for the child. It has long been known that, for all of us, cortisol levels vary through the day, peaking around waking-up time. On top of the constant high cortisol levels in children from trauma, this peak can cause quite severe symptoms. For many of them, every morning they 'wake up to war', feeling disorientated and panicky and ready to fight.

There are many things to try when dealing with this difficult time, described in 'Strategies for Waking Early/Angry' in *The A–Z* (Naish 2018, p.282).

Further strategies

These may be given to parents to aid the development of object permanence:

- *Give them a photograph of you* to take to school. A photo on a keyring or in the child's bag or pocket will be a visual reminder of your existence during the school day.
- *Something that smells of you* can help; this can be either your natural smell or a perfume or aftershave you habitually wear. We know that smell is extremely helpful when building the bonds of attachment. Maybe the child could take something that smells of you to bed with them, perhaps the t-shirt or cardigan that you've been wearing that day.
- *A bear or soft toy* with your voice recorded inside can be comforting. This is particularly helpful for younger children as they can press the bear at any time and hear your reassuring voice.
- *Give them your itinerary* while they are at school. We need to remember that many of our children have actually been removed and taken into care or moved to another family within the care system from school. Some of our children are very concerned that you will not be collecting them at the end of the day. Further to this, where a child has lived with domestic abuse they can be extremely worried about the wellbeing of parents whilst at school. This could also be said for children whose parents have chronic addictions. The itinerary assures them of what you're doing whilst they are at school.
- *Draw a heart on your wrist and the child's wrist*, agreeing to press the heart at numerous times during the day, letting the child know you will be thinking of them. You can also use an invisible string analogy, which works just as well.
- *The invisible hug.* This is where the parent will give the child a hug in the morning on their way to school, asking the child to look after the hug all day so they can give it back to the parent in the evening. It was actually a foster parent I worked with who shared this strategy with me, and it's been very helpful to many parents (see 'Separation Anxiety' in *The A–Z*, Naish 2018, pp.261–263).
- *Play games* such as peek-a-boo and hide-and-seek. These can also be helpful with older children, but we may need to adapt them somewhat. Other games can also help: guessing which little pot a ball is under is useful, as revealing the ball after moving the pots around is evidence that things continue to exist when you can't see them. Pelmanism, the game in which cards are spread, face down, and players pick up two, looking for a matching pair and replacing them in the same position if they don't match, does the same, with the added benefit of exercising memory.

Combining some or all of these strategies will help a child to begin to develop object permanence quite quickly, and many of the parents I've worked with have stated that they can see an improvement in behaviours associated with a lack of object permanence in just a few weeks.

CORNERSTONE 3: REGULAR RELATIONSHIP REPAIRS

Cornerstone explained

When laying the third cornerstone for children from trauma we must first understand the role of shame.

Shame is a developmental stage experienced by toddlers. It is the ugly feeling a child gets when corrected or disciplined by a parent or caregiver. This discipline is in the form of limits set by parents to aid child socialization and to curtail dangerous or negative behaviour. When a child experiences shame it deactivates the sympathetic nervous system and activates the parasympathetic nervous system. The child may cover their face, hide, shrink or burst into tears. They feel very uncomfortable when experiencing shame as it can signal a break in the relationship with their primary caregiver.

Securely attached children move relatively quickly through this stage and go on to develop healthy guilt, compassion, empathy and a conscience. This process is facilitated by the parent or caregiver who quickly repairs any relationship fracture. The parent will soothe and regulate the child and remind them that they are still loved, good, etc.

This enables the child to differentiate between themselves and their behaviour. They begin to internalize the knowledge that the relationship with their parent is intact and unconditional. Their internal working model is positive; they believe they are good, loveable, worthy and safe.

In essence, shame says 'I am a bad person' and guilt says 'What I've done is wrong'. All children should believe that they are intrinsically good whilst acknowledging right from wrong behaviour.

Unfortunately, children with a history of trauma and neglect have a limited experience of relationship repair, and sadly, some have none. Many have been punished and shunned and are therefore stuck in relationship rupture with their primary attachment figure.

This constant state of relationship rupture produces toxic shame within the child. They view themselves as bad, disgusting, unloveable, unworthy and as a failure.

The feeling of self-disgust is overwhelming, all-encompassing and often soul-destroying. This unmet developmental need will remain unmet without regular relationship repair. The repair can be extremely difficult for many parents and caregivers as behaviours exhibited by the child are often contrary to their own moral code.

Associated presenting behaviours

Sarah (Naish 2018, p.25) describes how children seek to avoid the feeling of shame:

If a child has not had their early, most basic needs met, they are consumed with a toxic form of shame. Our children work hard to stay out of this shame because it is truly devastating and all consuming. Some of the behaviours we see that relate to shame avoidance are:

- Lying
- An inability to take responsibility
- Self-sabotage.

Other behaviours closely associated with shame include the following:

- Stealing.
- Blaming others.
- Minimizing their behaviour.
- Defensive rage.
- Control and defiance.

Further to this, the child will actively but unconsciously seek rejection, physical punishment, removal of possessions, grounding, loss of privileges and time out. This is because the child is conditioned to believe that this is what to expect from adults and from life in general. The child feels comfortable when treated this way as this is what they are used to. Sadly such standard parenting approaches, frequently championed by unskilled supporting professionals, 'fit' the child's negative internal working model and confirm what they already believe to be true about themselves.

REWARD CHARTS
This is why reward charts absolutely do not work for children with a history of trauma and neglect. They are a visual reminder of the ways in which the children view themselves as bad.

Because of this, reward charts actually do harm by entrenching the behaviour that is a communication of their internal distress rather than deliberate naughtiness or defiance. Reward charts and reward schemes set the child up to fail: the good behaviour is often unachievable due to toxic shame and living in a constant fight, flight or freeze state.

In Chapter 6 of *The A–Z* Sarah explains why therapeutic parents avoid using reward charts (Naish 2018, p.61) and clearly outlines the reasons (Naish 2018, pp.244–245). The following are relevant here:

We don't use standard reward charts with children who have a background of trauma. There are several reasons for this:

- They can cause conflict with the child's internal working model – the child then chooses to stay on the 'bad side' to prove they are not worthy, or that they do not care.
- The child believes they are 'bad' in any case, so seeing other children succeeding reinforces their sense of failure and 'badness'.
- The child quickly learns to exploit reward charts, making them redundant.
- The child learns really fast how to manipulate the reward system to get the reward they need with minimum effort.
- Basic reward charts don't tackle most of the underlying entrenched behaviours and cannot take account of impulsivity and lack of cause-and-effect thinking.

The child's negative internal working model will also invariably lead to sabotage of fun and enjoyable times. The children do not believe that they deserve to experience joy and often feel bad and unworthy when they have done so.

This is compounded for children in care, who may feel they have been disloyal to their birth parents by engaging in a fun activity with their caregiver.

Many parents have described situations where they have taken a child out and had a wonderful time, only for a significant deterioration in behaviour later on that day. In addition, parents report that their children will often sabotage birthdays, Christmas and parties. Many will break or destroy their belongings, pictures or drawings as they cannot cope with praise or don't believe they deserve nice things.

Sarah (Naish 2018, pp.244–245) clearly outlines the reasons behind such behaviour:

- Comfortable to be 'in the wrong' – the child's internal working model convinces them they do not deserve nice things. This creates conflict within the child.
- Blocked trust – the child does not trust the honesty or motivation of the person providing the positive praise or gift or event.
- Recreating a familiar environment – the child is unfamiliar with receiving nice things or being given special time and/or has witnessed a disregard for property and personal appearance.
- Lack of cause-and-effect thinking – not able to remember that if something is broken, it stays broken.
- Dysregulation – acting in the heat of the moment.
- Shame – relating to feelings of unworthiness.
- Feelings of hostility or momentary hatred towards the parent.
- Loyalty to birth parents/former carers – resisting attachment to new carers/parents.

The child is stuck in this cycle of behaviours and has little or no empathy for others or for their future selves.

In the 'Introduction' to *The A–Z*, Sarah describes the child's lack of empathy:

Empathy is usually one of the last skills to develop. Our children need to have all their basic needs met before they can build on those and develop the more profound human characteristics such as empathy, gratitude and remorse. I have found that in general, children who have suffered trauma in early life need to have been responded to empathically, as in 'modelled empathy', for about seven to ten years before they can start to genuinely experience and demonstrate it. (Naish 2018, p.22)

In extreme cases children and young adults who are drowning in toxic shame will smear faeces, self-harm or actively seek removal from their current home.

Further to this, shame can cause children to frequently become irrationally angry with others, sometimes resorting to overtly aggressive and destructive actions. Understandably, those caring for these children will struggle to access empathy when such behaviours are often extreme and relentless.

In light of the above, we need to remain alert for symptoms of compassion fatigue in parents who are caring for children from trauma. Further information and advice around self-care and recognizing and managing compassion fatigue can be found in Chapter 7 in *The A–Z* (Naish 2018, pp.68–74) and also within our research into compassion fatigue (Ottaway and Selwyn 2016).

Therapeutic parenting approach and strategies

Therapeutic parenting helps parents to begin to depersonalize these behaviours and recognize them as a mode of communication. An awareness of the underlying emotion and unmet need for relationship consistency becomes the focus for the therapeutic parent and enables them to remain empathic and connected.

The open and engaged parent can then offer genuine relationship repair as they consciously respond to this unmet developmental need as opposed to emotionally reacting to the presenting behaviours.

It is important that the therapeutic parent is continually aware of their own internal triggers as this awareness will dilute the intensity of an emotional reaction in the moment. Effective therapeutic parenting begins with the parent's own ability to self-regulate. An internal dialogue within the parent enables them to evaluate, reflect, depersonalize and connect, even when faced with extremely challenging situations. Here are some useful phrases to use with a therapeutic parent:

Evaluate: Is this a shame-based behaviour?

Reflect: What is this behaviour triggering in the parent?

Depersonalize: Remember, the behaviour arises from shame; it is not personal

Connect: Think 'toddler'. Repair the relationship and remind the child they are still loved and cared for

Standard parenting leans towards issuing a consequence for the behaviour prior to the relationship repair. This is managed well by the securely attached child as they have internalized their primary attachment figure and are certain of relationship constancy. However, this is not the case for children and young people who have experienced ruptured attachments and little, if any, relationship repair.

The therapeutic parent repairs the rupture immediately, letting the child know that they are safe, loved, cared for and remaining with them prior to implementing a consequence. This process cannot effectively be carried out if the parent is dysregulated, but must take place as soon as the parent or caregiver feels calm again, otherwise the relationship remains in rupture and the child's toxic shame increases. This can quickly escalate into a further deterioration of behaviour and affirm the child's negative internal working model.

Asking or insisting that children say sorry arises from our own need to hear the word and move on from our own uncomfortable feelings. The child doesn't actually 'feel' sorry and will often comply only to end the conflict and access the next thing they want. In order to reduce shame and help them to link cause and effect, parents and caregivers need to encourage them to 'show sorry'. This can be an act of service for the person they've upset, hurt or offended, for example making a drink for someone, rubbing cream into the parent's arm etc. if they've hurt them, washing up, sweeping leaves, or something similar.

Responses and strategies to avoid can be found in Chapter 6 in *The A–Z* (Naish 2018, pp.59–67).

In order to strengthen attachment, it is beneficial if the child does something 'with' the parent and is thanked afterwards.

Writing letters or cards of apology is not advisable as the child will often sit in a 'pool of shame' whilst writing them, or simply just lie to get it out of the way.

Think of a time you have upset someone and that awful feeling you have until you put things right. The sense of relief is enormous. Now imagine having that feeling of shame *all* of the time! When children are offered an opportunity to repair by 'showing sorry', the toxic shame begins to reduce, and this particular incident is less likely to be added to their huge list of reasons that they're bad, unloveable and unworthy.

Sarah explains:

Our children are very unlikely to be able to feel remorse and give any kind of meaningful apology. Instead, we help our children to 'show sorry'. Our children usually do want to put right what they have done wrong, but they don't know how to. We might say, 'Oh I see you have tipped your sister's juice on the floor. Here is a cloth so you can help me clear it up.' Then afterwards give positive reinforcement. (Naish 2018, p.55)

Dismantling shame takes a long time and is hard work, but a constant awareness of it can enable parents to seek ways to challenge the negative self-belief the child holds and help them to view themselves through a new and more positive lens.

Sarah describes sabotaging in detail in Part 2 of *The A–Z* (2018, pp.244–249). The following are the most applicable to this particular cornerstone:

- *Do not over-praise or use general praise.* Be specific, but phrase carefully from your experience of the child. For example you may decide that saying 'That's an interesting drawing; I like the colours' is safer than 'I like your choice of colours' as the latter risks the child destroying the drawing because in their mind they are bad, so the choice must be bad (see p.63 of *The A–Z*).
- *Low-key birthdays.* The child intrinsically believes that the only impact they have ever had on the world is a negative one, and that includes being born. This is another aspect of their negative internal working model. Although they may appear to want to celebrate their birthday, they have an internal conflict with this belief. Keeping it low key makes it easier for them to manage and they are thus less likely to sabotage it (see pp.103–106 of *The A–Z*).

- *Low-key Christmas.* Christmas is a time when families celebrate together, and it can therefore trigger feelings of unworthiness, disloyalty and rejection. Children with a negative internal working model will sometimes refuse to play with or destroy expensive gifts because they believe they don't deserve them (see pp.103–106 of *The A–Z*).
- *Good heart.* Encourage parents to remind the child that they have a good heart by pointing out examples of this, because without evidence, they won't believe it. For example, if they take the parent's cup out to the kitchen, the parent might say: 'Thank you – I knew you had a good heart.' Parents need to be careful to do this in a light-hearted way and then swiftly move on. This helps them internalize it without reacting to it (see, for example, p.248 of *The A–Z*).
- *Avoid saying 'no'.* Due to the child's negative internal working model, they do not hear us saying 'no' to something they want. Sadly, the 'no' that they hear means 'no' to them as a person rather than to the thing that they want. It catapults them into shame and can trigger defensive rage. It is far more helpful for a parent to say something like: 'I can see you really want to play with your toys but we're going to school now. You can play with your toys when you get home.' Using positive responses will reduce shame and keep the relationship with the parent intact throughout, even when the child is defiant.
- *Acceptance and empathy.* Parents need to accept and acknowledge a child's feelings of inadequacy, shame and unworthiness, and empathize with these feelings; note, however, that empathizing does not mean agreeing. An example would be if a child said that they were bad and horrible – telling them that they were good and not to feel that way would leave the child feeling not heard and misunderstood. Therefore parents need to say something like: 'Wow! It must be really difficult to feel that way. I need to work hard to help you to see what I see' (see, for example, 'Acceptance' on p.53 of *The A–Z* and 'Empathy' on pp.14 and 45–46).

The aim here is to give the child a different lens through which to view themselves and to demonstrate to them that the relationship with their parent or caregiver is unconditional and unaffected by their behaviour. It may take a long time for a parent to see a significant improvement in shame-based behaviours. However, consistent responding in such a way will progressively dilute the child's negative internal working model and help them to develop healthy guilt, empathy, compassion and a conscience.

CORNERSTONE 4: LINKING CAUSE AND EFFECT

Cornerstone explained

The only way a new-born baby can communicate is through behaviour, notably crying, turning their head away, pulling their legs up or making sucking movements. They enter into the arousal–relaxation cycle with their primary caregiver and their communicated needs are interpreted and met. The baby is then conditioned to believe that there is a connection between what they do and getting their needs met. The baby starts to believe that they are having a positive influence on their environment.

By seven or eight months they are beginning to experiment with anything to hand, such as toys, moving and manipulating them to see what happens. This is further development of their experience of cause and effect, which deepens and widens as the baby grows. Even the seemingly aimless arm waving is part of this learning: they are training their hand–eye coordination ('When my arm feels like this, it's over here').

Cause-and-effect learning becomes increasingly specific with age, so, for example, the toddler learns that if they hit their tower of bricks, it falls over. In learning these lessons, predictability and consistency are necessary. With these two, the world then becomes predictable.

The child understands that there is a consequence to their actions, and they begin to realize that they can determine the outcome by choosing the appropriate behaviour. They are able to pause, evaluate and reflect before acting.

A child who has experienced trauma and neglect has not been able to learn these lessons. This is not just a nebulous idea: the necessary physical brain development has not taken place, and the evidence can be seen in brain scans, for example those obtained by Dr Bruce D. Perry, Senior Fellow of the Child Trauma Academy in Houston, Texas, and an Adjunct Professor of Psychiatry and Behavioral Sciences at the Feinberg School of Medicine in Chicago, Illinois, USA.

In the 'Introduction' to *The A–Z* Sarah explains that therapeutic parenting is used to address this deficit:

> The aim of therapeutic parenting is to enable the child to recover from the trauma they have experienced. This is done by developing new pathways in the child's brain to help them to link cause and effect, reduce their levels of fear and shame, and to help them start to make sense of their world. (Naish 2018, p.13)

Because the baby's arousal–relaxation cycle, which is based on trust and security that an adult will respond to their needs, was inadequate, and because of the aforementioned negative internal working model, the baby is conditioned to believe that their impact on the world is negative.

For some children, one meal did not follow another, their life did not follow the cycle of night and day, and they had no predictability whatsoever. They are trapped in a constant state of survival; the reasoning part of their brain is underdeveloped and what does exist is mostly unavailable to them.

In Chapter 1 of *The A–Z*, Sarah states:

> Where our children have suffered some kind of trauma in their lives, nothing is predictable. Their early lives may have made no sense. My children did not know the difference between night and day. If even the basics of human existence make no sense, then it is much harder for the more complex layers to be ordered into a fathomable structure by these children. As the children tend to act quickly on impulse, without forward planning, they often suffer as a direct result of their own actions. This is because many of our own inhibitors stem from the fact that we don't want to feel bad later. For example, we might not steal £10 from the kitchen table because we know we might get in trouble, or we don't want to feel bad. Our children cannot project forward and think about how they might feel later. In effect, they lack empathy for their future self. (Naish 2018, p.21)

Associated presenting behaviours

What behaviours may we see as a result of a deficit in cause-and-effect thinking?

- Acting on impulse.
- Not considering how their behaviour affects either themselves or other people.
- Not thinking about the consequence of their behaviour.
- Inability to project themselves into the future and predict an outcome.
- Unable to learn via punitive consequences, for example standard parenting interventions such as time out, naughty step, loss of privileges, being lectured to, etc.
- Not trusting in the predictability of one event following another.

As already noted, all these things are typical of the average toddler, and we therefore need to ask ourselves how toddlers move beyond these, and how we can help a chronologically older child to do so.

The starting point is establishing the parent as the unassailable safe base – the first cornerstone.

The use of the visual timetable described under the first cornerstone also helps to develop cause-and-effect thinking because the child can see what follows what.

Therapeutic parenting approach and strategies

Both natural and logical consequences are key here, not least because they are the ways in which most toddlers learn of the impact of their own actions.

Natural consequences are those that happen without the intervention of the parent. For example, if I run in the rain without shoes I get wet feet, if I don't wear a coat I get cold, and if I break my toy it doesn't work anymore.

Logical consequences are put in place by the parent, and they are as a result of a choice the child has made. For example, if I hit my parent on the arm, it becomes painful and my parent then can't drive me to Youth Club.

I remember my foster mum continually nagging me, to no avail, to brush my teeth. I would either flatly refuse or become argumentative. One day she responded by 'sadly' stating that it would be such a shame if I couldn't have ice cream later that day as unfortunately you can't put sugar on dirty teeth. I soon brushed them!

In Chapter 3 of *The A–Z*, Sarah explains natural consequences thus:

Natural consequences are the life consequences that follow, usually when a boundary is broken or the child has made a bad choice. We set our boundaries and then, when they are breached – usually through immaturity and the lack of cause-and-effect thinking – we show our children that they have made an impact on the world, through natural consequences with nurture. If we fail to do that we are setting us all up to fail in the long run. We are reinforcing the message that the child's actions are of no consequence.

I used natural consequences to build synapses in my child's brain, which linked cause and effect, and the world started to make sense to them.

Natural consequences must be used with nurture. It is sometimes too tempting to over-punish the child through manipulating consequences and calling them natural consequences. (Naish 2018, p.39)

Visual timetables can help specifically with logical consequences concerning lost time for an activity they enjoy. For example, a child refusing to put their toys away before lunch means that lunch is delayed and thus there is less time at the park later. The child learns that their actions affect both their own world and the world of others.

For the child to learn the lesson it is not necessary to match minute for minute, and doing so risks fracturing the relationship and becoming punitive. It is enough that the child loses some time at the park, and it can be however much fits best into the rest of the schedule.

It is crucial that the parent empathizes with the child while they are experiencing these consequences because the relationship between them needs to remain intact throughout. If not, the child falls into the shame pit and the lesson is lost. For example, the parent might say, 'I know it's difficult for you and it's such a shame we don't have as much time at the park, so let's make the most of the time we do have.'

In Chapter 6 of *The A–Z*, Sarah explains the futility of consequences that are unrelated to the child's behaviour (Naish 2018, pp.63–64).

Natural and logical consequences actually build and/or strengthen synapses in the brain, and a lack of these new connections is what shows up on the brain scans referred to above. There are lots of examples of natural consequences relating to specific challenges in *The A–Z*.

THE DEVELOPMENTAL FOUNDATION PLANNER – JOSH

The Developmental Foundation Planner is a series of tables, all but one of which is filled in for each individual child.

The first function of the tool is to indicate which of the cornerstones is in most need of strengthening. Or, to put it another way, where can we most effectively concentrate our efforts in order to meet unmet developmental needs?

This example is based on Josh when he is five years old and has been with his therapeutic foster parent Linda for six months. Linda is a single parent and regularly helps to care for her two-year-old grandson Tom while his parents are at work.

Linda has noticed that, although Josh is chronologically age five, he appears to be developmentally on a par with Tom, and she raised this with her supervising social worker, Emma, during a recent supervision. Because Linda has had the relevant training she is aware that this is symptomatic of Developmental Trauma Disorder, but she needs some guidance around how to respond to and meet Josh's unmet developmental needs. Emma suggests using the Developmental Foundation Planner.

Emma alerts both Glynis, Linda's empathic listener, and the fostering agency attachment therapist Julie, who arranges a meeting with Linda and Emma to gain an overview of Josh's current behaviours and how these relate to his unmet developmental needs.

Table 1 is generic. It shows, for each cornerstone, behaviours that can arise from weakness in a cornerstone. As such, it enables everyone to identify which of Josh's behaviours arise from which of his unmet developmental needs and, thus, which cornerstone needs strengthening first. It is crucial to note that any weakness in cornerstone 1 must be addressed before any of the others can be successfully tackled. Furthermore, if a child has a deficit in cornerstone 1, they will definitely have deficits in the other three cornerstones.

Table 1. Behaviours that can arise from weaknesses in each cornerstone

Cornerstone 1: Establishing the parent as the unassailable safe base	Cornerstone 2: Developing object permanence	Cornerstone 3: Regular relationship repairs	Cornerstone 4: Linking cause and effect
Avoiding adults to keep safe	Following	Lying	Acting on impulse
Befriending adults to keep safe	Incessant chatter	Stealing	Not considering how their behaviour affects either themselves or other people
Not asking for help	Nonsense questions	Blaming others	Not thinking about the consequence of their behaviour
Fake smiling	Fear of invisibility	Denying responsibility	Inability to project themselves into the future and predict an outcome
Hiding in their bedroom	Fear of being forgotten	Defensive rage	Can't learn via punitive consequences, e.g. time out, naughty step, loss of privileges, being lectured to, etc.
Anxious and clingy	Fear of the adult leaving their presence	Controlling and defiant	
Saying that everything is fine when it's not	Frequent need to check availability of the adult	Actively but unconsciously seeking rejection, physical punishment, removal of possessions, grounding, loss of privileges and time out	
Unable to genuinely access adults for comfort and co-regulation	Repeatedly saying 'hello' to an adult when they reappear after a brief absence	Sabotaging birthdays, Christmas and parties	
Not trusting adults to meet their needs	Problems going to sleep	Sabotaging fun	
Innate need to be in control	Frequent waking	Breaking or destroying their belongings, pictures or drawings	
Believing that it is only a matter of time before they are moved on	Calling out in the night	Smearing and/or urinating in places other than the toilet	

People-pleasing	Difficulty remaining in their bedroom	Self-harming	
Rejecting adults	Dysregulation at school	Actively seeking removal from current home	
Lack of sense of belonging	Cannot delay gratification	Irrational anger	
Failing to follow instructions from an adult		Aggressive	
Failing to follow instructions from an adult whilst pretending to do so		Destructive	
Overly compliant			
Secretive			
Withdrawn and insular			
Disingenuous and inauthentic (masking)			
Cannot self-regulate			
Pretending to share the adult's interests			
Aggressive			
Destructive			
Violent			

From looking at Table 1, Linda was quickly able to see that Josh has not yet established her as his unassailable safe base and hasn't experienced regular relationship repairs. Emma and Julie helped Linda to complete Table 2, which sets out Josh's known history and his presenting behaviours. Much of this information was gathered from the Trauma Tracker, which had already been completed for Josh.

Table 2 has been completed for Josh. 'History/chronology' here means the parts of Josh's known history that help to identify his unmet developmental needs. Column 1 contains specific events or experiences and column 2 the consequential unmet developmental needs and associated trauma responses. Column 3 gives *The A–Z* page reference applicable to column 2, and is only here for the purposes of this book. Columns 4–7 are for the four cornerstones, and a tick indicates where the cornerstone is related to the specific information in column 2.

Once completed, the ticks are tallied up, and cornerstones needing the most attention are identified.

Table 2. Josh's known history

History/ chronology	Consequential unmet developmental needs and associated trauma responses	*The A–Z* reference page(s)	Cornerstone 1: Establishing the parent as the unassailable safe base	Cornerstone 2: Developing object permanence	Cornerstone 3: Regular relationship repairs	Cornerstone 4: Linking cause and effect
Mother highly stressed and anxious throughout the pregnancy because of domestic abuse and homelessness	Not claimed during pregnancy	32–39, Chapter 3: 'The Essential Foundations of Therapeutic Parenting'	☐			
	Unsuitable in utero environment due to flooding with the stress hormone cortisol, so 'wired for danger' when born	26–27: 'Sensory issues'	✓			
	Unable to enter into a healthy attachment cycle	18–19: 'The car driver'	✓	✓		✓
	Not developing a positive internal working model	25–26: 'The child's internal working model'	✓			✓
Very little nurturing attention from his biological mother	Not building a secure attachment	18–19: 'The car driver'	✓		✓	
	No available adult	21: 'Blocked trust'	✓	✓		✓
	Lack of predictability	18–19: 'The car driver'	✓	✓		✓
	No routine, structure or healthy boundaries	37–38: 'Establish strong clear boundaries'	✓	✓	✓	✓
	Lack of affection	46–47: 'Nurture'	✓		✓	
	Little experience of co-regulation	53–54: 'Use touch and parental presence to regulate'	✓		✓	

Experience	Impact	Reference				
Left alone in the home	Feeling abandoned and unsafe	23–24: 'Fear of invisibility'	✓	✓	✓	
	Underdeveloped sense of object permanence	23–24: 'Fear of invisibility'	✓	✓		
	Insufficient access to food and drink	27: 'Interoception'	✓			✓
No one got up to him in the night	Underdeveloped sense of object permanence	23–24: 'Fear of invisibility'	✓	✓	✓	✓
	Feeling abandoned	23–24: 'Fear of invisibility'	✓	✓		
Shouted and screamed at a lot	Shame	45: 'Empathize'	✓		✓	
	Toxic shame	45: 'Empathize'	✓		✓	
	No regular relationship repairs	20: 'Unable to re-attune'	✓		✓	
	Negative internal working model embedded	25–26: 'The child's internal working model'	✓		✓	
	Fear of adults	20: 'Fear'	✓		✓	
Ignored	Feeling invisible	23–24: 'Fear of invisibility'	✓	✓		
	Fear of being forgotten	23–24: 'Fear of invisibility'	✓	✓		
	Not learned to play	179–182: 'Immaturity'	✓			✓
	Shame	45: 'Empathize'	✓		✓	
	Fear of dying	20: 'Fear'	✓			
Physically abused	Unsafe	20: 'Fear'	✓			
	Fear of adults	20: 'Fear'	✓		✓	
	Toxic shame	45: 'Empathize'	✓		✓	
	Physical pain	27: 'Interoception'	✓			
	Traumatic explicit and implicit memories	25–26: 'The child's internal working model'	✓			

History/ chronology	Consequential unmet developmental needs and associated trauma responses	The A–Z reference page(s)	Cornerstone 1: Establishing the parent as the unassailable safe base	Cornerstone 2: Developing object permanence	Cornerstone 3: Regular relationship repairs	Cornerstone 4: Linking cause and effect
Insufficient and inadequate food	Hunger	27: 'Interoception'	✓			✓
	Fear of food being unavailable	150–155: 'Food Issues'	✓	✓		✓
	Unpredictability	38–39: 'The car driver'	✓	✓		✓
Surrounded by dangerous adults	Fear of dying	20: 'Fear'	✓		✓	
	Toxic shame	45: 'Empathize'	✓		✓	
	Unpredictability	38–39: 'Use natural (or life) consequences'	✓			✓
Witnessed domestic abuse	Unsafe	20: 'Fear'	✓		✓	
	Fear of adults	20: 'Fear'	✓		✓	
	Toxic shame	45: 'Empathize'	✓		✓	
	Physical pain	27: 'Interoception'	✓			
	Traumatic explicit and implicit memories	25–26: 'The child's internal working model'	✓			
Witnessed adults abusing drugs and alcohol	Unsafe	20: 'Fear'	✓			
	Fear of adults	20: 'Fear'	✓		✓	
	Toxic shame	45: 'Empathize'	✓		✓	
	Physical pain	27: 'Interoception'	✓			
	Traumatic explicit and implicit memories	25–26: 'The child's internal working model'	✓			

No routine	No consistency, predictability or reliable adults	38–39: 'Use natural (or life) consequences'	✓	✓	✓	✓
	Underdeveloped sense of object permanence	23–24: 'Fear of invisibility'	✓	✓		
	Cannot link cause and effect	38–39: 'Use natural (or life) consequences'				✓
Hygiene needs unmet	Unclean; cannot wash or dress self; not adequately toilet trained	93–96: 'Bath Time Issues'	✓		✓	
Medical and dental needs unmet	Possible undiagnosed medical conditions	33–35: 'Establish yourself as the unassailable safe base'	✓		✓	
	Not had all the necessary vaccinations	33–35: 'Establish yourself as the unassailable safe base'	✓			
Educational needs unmet	Academically behind	249–256: 'School Issues'	✓		✓	✓
No toys	Cannot play	179–182: 'Immaturity'	✓			
Numerous house moves	No consistency or predictability	38–39: 'Use natural (or life) consequences'	✓		✓	✓
	No safe base to call home	33–35: 'Establish yourself as the unassailable safe base'	✓	✓		
Total ticks			55	15	25	16

After completing Table 2, everybody had a very clear picture of how Josh's history offered much insight into his unmet developmental needs. Linda was correct in her belief that Josh had not established a parent as his unassailable safe base in early childhood and that he was flooded with shame due to constant relationship rupture with his primary caregivers.

Linda explained that completing this table had helped her to further understand Josh, and things were now beginning to make a lot of sense.

Linda, Julie and Emma then completed Table 3. Table 3 looks at Josh's current behaviours and identifies the correlating cornerstone. A tick indicates where the cornerstone is related to the behaviours described in column 1.

In Table 3 below, column 2 is only included for the purposes of this book.

Table 3. Josh's current presenting behaviours

Current presenting behaviours	*The A–Z* reference page(s)	Cornerstone 1: Establishing the parent as the unassailable safe base	Cornerstone 2: Developing object permanence	Cornerstone 3: Regular relationship repairs	Cornerstone 4: Linking cause and effect
Violence	81–86	✓		✓	
Swearing	305–307	✓		✓	
Cannot settle at school	249–256	✓	✓		
Speaking in a baby voice	179–182	✓			
Cannot play	182	✓			✓
Sleep issues	96–99 (bedtime) 277–283 (sleep)	✓	✓		✓
Befriends men	115–118	✓			
Struggles to be around women	20 (fear)	✓			
Defiance	134–137	✓		✓	
Cannot self-regulate	53–54	✓		✓	
Doesn't think about the consequences of his behaviour	38–39	✓			✓
Jealous of Linda's grandson Tom	273–277	✓		✓	
Preoccupied with food	150–155	✓	✓		✓

Runs away	77–80	✓		✓	✓
Cannot bear to be told 'no'	25–26 (shame)	✓		✓	
Needs to be in control	124–128	✓		✓	
Total ticks		**16**	**3**	**8**	**5**

Completing Table 3 gave very similar results to those from Table 2, that is, the historical chronology and the behaviour both indicate the same prioritization of unmet needs. This is particularly useful because it allows a child's needs to be identified even when the historical record is incomplete or absent.

Julie added together the totals from Tables 2 and 3 to gather an overall total for unmet developmental needs applicable to the cornerstones from Josh's known historical chronology and those communicated via his behaviour. The results are shown in Table 4.

Table 4. Accumulative totals from Tables 2 and 3

Totals	Cornerstone 1	Cornerstone 2	Cornerstone 3	Cornerstone 4
Table 2	55	15	25	16
Table 3	16	3	8	5
Overall total	**71**	**18**	**33**	**21**

The overall totals gave Julie, Emma and Linda the necessary information for identifying which cornerstones to concentrate on. They were aware that *all* cornerstones need addressing, but they now felt they at least had a starting point.

Completing Tables 2 and 3 helped to identify that cornerstones 1 and 3 needed urgent attention, although cornerstones 2 and 4 would also be taken into consideration when planning the necessary approach and strategies for Josh. This is because, just as in a house, all four cornerstones are needed.

Together they proceeded to complete Tables 5–8, one for each cornerstone, in the order of priority (number of ticks in Table 4). Thus Table 5 is for Cornerstone 1, Table 6 for Cornerstone 3, and so on.

In each table, column 1 lists the particular behaviours exhibited by Josh under the relevant cornerstones and column 2 details suggested strategies specific to Josh's needs.

Approach

Josh's history indicates that he has never experienced an adult as an unassailable safe base. This means he will not have been adequately claimed as a baby and will have extreme fear of adults. He will not trust an adult's motives and will believe they cannot meet his needs and will not keep him safe. For this reason, it is vitally important that Linda keeps this information at the forefront of her mind at all times when responding to Josh.

Claiming him is essential, as are warm and nurturing responses throughout. Further to this, Linda must be in charge. She cannot allow Josh to make the decisions about what is happening but can empathize with him when he resists. Lots of playful responses will also be highly beneficial. Using a warm and empathic tone of voice will reduce some of his fear and anxiety.

Table 5. Cornerstone 1: Establishing the parent as the unassailable safe base

Exhibited associated behaviours	Suggested strategies from the list in the Developmental Foundation Planner
Aggression and violence	Boundaries
	Routine and structure
	Empathic commentary
	Parental presence
Swearing	Boundaries
Cannot settle at school	'Naming the need'
	Visual timetable
Speaking in a baby voice	Empathic commentary
	Claiming vocabulary
Cannot play	Play with the child at developmental or emotional stage
	Use toys and games for younger children
Sleep issues	Visual timetable
	Routine
	Empathic commentary
	Staying close or parental presence
Befriends men	Empathic commentary
	'Naming the need'
Struggles to be around women	Empathic commentary
	'Naming the need'
Defiant	Visual timetable
	Routine or structure
	Boundaries
Cannot self-regulate	Claiming the child using a claiming vocabulary and empathic commentary
	Staying close
Doesn't think about the consequences of his behaviour	Empathic commentary
	Routine
Jealous of Linda's grandson Tom	Claiming the child using a claiming vocabulary and empathic commentary

Preoccupied with food	'Naming the need'
	Routine
	Visual timetable
Runs away	Staying close or parental presence
	Empathic commentary
Cannot bear to be told 'no'	Empathic commentary
	Boundaries
Needs to be in control	Routine
	Structure
	Boundaries
	Parent in charge

Approach

Tables 2 and 3 clearly indicate that Josh has high levels of toxic shame and a negative internal working model. His history shows that he has been physically and emotionally abused which unfortunately has further embedded his belief that he is a 'bad' child. This is why it is of paramount importance that Linda endeavours to keep their relationship intact throughout any incidents, particularly violent ones. The violence he displays arises from defensive rage due to extreme shame. Therefore, any relationship ruptures must be followed by an immediate repair before implementing a consequence, if one is needed.

Table 6. Cornerstone 3: Regular relationship repairs

Exhibited associated behaviours	Suggested strategies from the list in the Developmental Foundation Planner
Aggression and violence	Good heart
	Acceptance and empathy
	Relationship repair
	'Showing sorry'
Swearing	Good heart
	Acceptance and empathy
	Relationship repair
Defiance	Empathic commentary
	Relationship repair
Cannot self-regulate	Keeping things low key
	Empathic commentary

Exhibited associated behaviours	Suggested strategies from the list in the Developmental Foundation Planner
Jealous of Linda's grandson Tom	Empathic commentary
	Acceptance and empathy
	Relationship repair
	'Showing sorry'
Runs away	Empathic commentary
	Relationship repair
Cannot bear to be told 'no'	Empathic commentary
	Boundaries
	Relationship repair
	Avoid using the word 'no'
Needs to be in control	Empathic commentary

Approach

Lack of routine and predictability in early life has severely impaired Josh's ability to link cause and effect. His needs were not adequately responded to and he struggles to understand how his behaviour affects an outcome. Linda needs to use natural and logical consequences with nurture and to remind Josh of what's happening next with the aid of a visual timetable.

Table 7. Cornerstone 4: Linking cause and effect

Exhibited associated behaviours	Suggested strategies from the list in the Developmental Foundation Planner
Cannot play	Visual timetable
	Natural consequences
Sleep issues	Visual timetable
	Logical consequences
Doesn't think about the consequences of his behaviour	Natural and logical consequences
Preoccupied with food	Visual timetables
Runs away	Natural and logical consequences

Approach

Josh did not have his needs met consistently and reliably as a baby, which means he hasn't fully developed object permanence. This has been compounded by the fact that he was left unsupervised and will have felt abandoned. Linda will need to take this into consideration whenever she is away from him. This is particularly relevant to his issues with school and sleeping.

Table 8. Cornerstone 2: Developing object permanence

Exhibited associated behaviours	Suggested strategies from the list in the Developmental Foundation Planner
Cannot settle at school	Empathic commentary
	Your itinerary
	Invisible hug
	Your photograph
Sleep issues	Getting up in the night
	Sand timers and singing
	Something that smells of you
Preoccupied with food	Visual timetable

Progress

Linda, Julie and Emma now had a plan of action, of which Glynis was informed. Julie and Emma observed that it would be hard work for Linda, but they were both there to support her. Linda felt more confident about her approach and found the tool had deepened her understanding of Josh's needs.

Two weeks later, Linda, Julie, Emma and Glynis met to discuss how things were going.

Linda said that she could already see some progress, particularly since she had begun to use claiming vocabulary and was sticking to the routine using a visual timetable. The most noticeable difference was that there had only been once incidence of violent behaviour in the fortnight.

Josh was still quite defiant and struggled with Linda sticking to the boundaries, but overall she had noticed an improvement in his behaviours. Josh had also asked for more hugs over the past week, which was quite unusual for him.

Table 9 tracks the progress. Column 1 lists Josh's presenting behaviours and a tick in column 2 indicates an improvement in these behaviours. Column 3 shows the most helpful strategies used by Linda to effect positive change. Column 4 details needs that are being met or addressed and column 5 suggests actions and strategies for those behaviours yet to improve. Where no action is indicated, Linda is to carry on using the same approach and strategies that have already proved helpful.

Note that 'Improved' doesn't mean the behaviours have dramatically reduced or ceased; it merely shows some improvement, even if only marginal.

Table 9. Progress tracking

Josh's exhibited behaviours	Improved?	Most helpful approach or strategies	Needs being met or addressed	Action or strategies agreed
Violence	✓	Claiming	Less fearful of Linda	
		Empathic commentary	Beginning to understand how his feelings link to his behaviour	
		Staying close or parental presence	Calms down more quickly	
		Natural and logical consequences	Helps to clean up any mess	
		Relationship repair	Open to connection with Linda	
Swearing	✓	Logical consequences	Linking cause and effect	
		Empathic commentary	Linking his behaviour to his feelings	
Cannot settle at school	✓	Linda's itinerary	Knows Linda is coming back	
		Linda's photograph on a keyring	Feeling claimed and wanted	
		Invisible hug	Nurture	
Speaking in a baby voice				Play and staying close, offering co-regulation
Cannot play				Play and using toys suitable for toddlers, including reading to him
Sleep issues	✓	Getting up in the night	Linda available at all times	
		Sand timer	Linking cause and effect Delaying gratification	
		Staying close or parental presence	Not abandoned	
		'Naming the need'	Understanding his own behaviour	
		Routine	Regulation and predictability	

Befriending men				Empathic commentary and staying close; co-regulation and 'naming the need'
Struggles to be around women				Empathic commentary and 'naming the need'
Defiance	✓	Empathic commentary	Josh starting to realize he swears more when he is dysregulated	
		Visual timetable	Linking cause and effect	
Cannot self-regulate				Staying close or parental presence and co-regulation
Doesn't think about the consequences of his behaviour	✓	Empathic commentary	Linking his behaviour to his feelings	
		Visual timetable	Linking cause and effect	
		Natural and logical consequences	Linking cause and effect	
Jealous of Linda's grandson Tom				Regular relationship repairs; empathic commentary and 'naming the need'
Preoccupied with food				Routine; visual timetable; 'naming the need'; empathic commentary
Runs away				Relationship repair; logical consequence; empathic commentary
Cannot bear to be told 'no'	✓	Avoiding using the word 'no'	Feels less shame Relationship remains intact	
Needs to be in control				Boundaries; empathic commentary

After completing Table 9, Linda said she felt that things were moving in the right direction, but was aware it was early days.

The team agreed to meet again in a month to reassess. Meanwhile, Glynis and Julie would keep in touch with Linda to offer support and guidance and Emma arranged weekly contact plus additional phone support whenever Linda needed her.

When the team met one month later they completed Table 9 again. There had been further improvement in all behaviours, and it was evident that all four cornerstones were being addressed. Linda said she felt tired but more hopeful about her ability to continue to meet Josh's unmet developmental needs using this tool.

The team agreed to meet at monthly intervals for a period of six months to continue to assess Josh's needs, but all supporting professionals offered their support and availability between meetings.

CONCLUSION

The Developmental Foundation Planner is a live tool, which means it is revisited as often as is deemed necessary for the individual child. I believe this tool is essential for all children from trauma, particularly for those adopted or in care. Ideally, it should be used as soon as a child comes into care, forming part of a child's care plan when placed with a family. This will help those caring for children from trauma to begin to meet unmet developmental needs as soon as a child moves in.

Meeting a child's unmet developmental needs alters the trajectory of their life and has the potential to interrupt the current devastating pattern of children from care having children who are also taken into care.

My foster mum did all she could to meet my unmet developmental needs and I'm truly grateful that as a result my own four children have never been in care and neither have my grandchildren. Thankfully, she knew that an unmet need remains unmet until it is met!

Part Three

Dousing the Sparks: The Behaviour – Assessment of Impact and Resolution Tool (BAIRT)

SARAH NAISH

This part will help readers to use an interactive assessment tool, the Behaviour – Assessment of Impact and Resolution Tool (BAIRT) – to identify issues as they arise that may threaten the stability of the family and the child. This is a step-by-step process that incorporates a guide to the assessment tool, how to use it and when. This is linked to Part 2 in *The A–Z* covering all the behaviours (Naish 2018).

THE IMPACT OF BEHAVIOURS FROM DEVELOPMENTAL TRAUMA

Trauma may be referred to as adverse childhood experiences (ACEs). The cause may be known about, that is, neglect or abuse, or it may stem from an as yet undiscovered event(s) or underlying condition. The important aspects we need to focus on in this intervention is to:

- Diminish or resolve the behaviours and their impact.
- Preserve and promote the evolving attachment between the child and their parent.
- Avoid unplanned moves and ruptures in the relationship.

In *The A–Z* I have written extensively about the behaviours that come from trauma, what they look like, why they happen and how to resolve the behaviours. *For this reason, the use of The A–Z alongside this Companion is an integral part of this intervention.*

The impact on parents who are caring for children from trauma cannot be underestimated. There is very little an unskilled professional can do (or perhaps even want to do) in the face of such overwhelming need and complex behaviours. Often supporting professionals will see that foster parents, adopters and other therapeutic parents begin to withdraw from the child they are caring for as a direct response to the level of difficult behaviours they are experiencing. This is normal.

In 2016 in our research we found that the impact of behaviours and the system on therapeutic parents or foster parents was significant (Ottaway and Selwyn 2016). Where there is compassion fatigue, parents withdraw. They may also become angry, resentful and scapegoat the child. It is at these times supporting professionals need to be confident and non-judgemental, and to draw closer to the family to help them to resolve the issues and to re-engage.

We can never do that from a position of high and mighty, blame and judgement!

Of course, this can be very difficult to balance in today's risk-averse, blame-fuelled social work culture. After all, our primary consideration is to protect the child, isn't it?

Yes, of course, but sometimes we do not see the full picture. Social workers have become accustomed to working in a way that reduces the likelihood of blame and assures short-term goals. The long-term impact is lost or minimized, and yet it is the *long-term impact* that is so vital and life-changing *for the child*. They don't get another chance at this.

HOW THE BAIRT WORKS

This tool supports an intervention which is designed to assist foster parents, adopters, other therapeutic parents *and* their professional supporters in identifying, understanding and improving or resolving difficult behaviours arising from children who have suffered trauma. It can also be used with birth parents where there are difficult presenting behaviours. Sometimes these behaviours might need adaptions made to the parenting style, and may help the parent and supporter in identifying other underlying issues and causative factors. For example, the impact of prenatal stress or domestic violence on a child who is living with birth parents may have been overlooked as a causative factor in presenting behaviours or issues such as sensory processing, etc.

Once we have established that the behaviours arising from developmental trauma are having a negative impact on the parent (and therefore the child), we need to:

- Assess the impact and severity of the behaviours.
- Design a bespoke intervention to resolve the impact and severity.
- Stabilize the family.

BAIRT helps the supporter to do this.

The supporter carrying out this assessment should be either a skilled supervising social worker, an empathic listener (that is, a skilled foster parent or adopter who has had similar experiences) or therapist (trained in Dyadic Developmental Psychotherapy, DDP, or similar) who is trusted by the parent, and able to feed back progress and seek support themselves from others in the team.

In families where there are two parents, the experience of both may well be different. In some families one parent may feel they are coping well and are not triggered by certain behaviours whilst another may feel overwhelmed by a difficult, repetitive behaviour. The supporter must first identify with whom they are working. Will it be both parents or just one? If both parents are taking part in the assessment, there will need to be a consensus about which behaviours (cornerstones) need to be focused on (see Part Two).

No direct work is undertaken with the child other than by the therapeutic parent.

WHEN TO USE THE BAIRT

During my time as a social worker and also running independent fostering agencies, I witnessed many situations where, when faced with a difficult behavioural challenge, the knee-jerk response of social workers was to blame and withdraw. This merely mimicked the actions and reactions within the family, and often led to avoidable disruption or removal of children.

Where there is developmental trauma and complex, relentless behaviours, social workers and other supporting professionals need to feel confident about dealing with these in a succinct, straightforward way of getting to the root of the behaviours and helping parents to resolve them in a supportive manner.

Often, situations are left to fester for too long. It can sometimes seem easier to ignore a difficult or complex challenge and hope it magically resolves itself. It rarely does!

In my therapeutic fostering agencies, I always get staff to be on the look-out for 'sparks'. Sparks are what we see when small changes or worrying patterns start to emerge. There might be escalations in defiance, controlling behaviours, absconding or aggression. If we leave these 'sparks' to go unchecked, they quickly multiply and become a fire. Where there is a fire, people often need to leave the building.

It is at times of crisis that parents turn to supporting professionals to help them with these tasks, yet ironically, it is these tasks that supporting professionals are often the least well equipped to deal with. Parents may also try to ignore the 'sparks' and to keep going far too long.

If we work proactively with parents and assure them that we are confident at dealing with the types of situations that they will face, we reassure them to report difficulties at an early stage, before situations become unmanageable. Good training and open conversations are essential to build mutual trust between therapeutic parents and supporting professionals.

The training needs to take place with staff and parents simultaneously in a culture of openness and mutual respect. Agencies and local authorities that separate out their foster parents or adopters from social workers (or worse still, only provide training for the parents) merely alienate the parents. The need for training in child trauma and therapeutic parenting is as important for social workers as it is for parents.

As a social worker I knew all about the legislation and how and when to remove a child. I learned very little about how to *keep* a child in a family and to resolve the challenges within it. Sadly, little seems to have changed in social work training today. Newly qualified social workers tell me that they have had virtually no training in childhood trauma and they leave university equipped only with a plethora of outdated traditional parenting techniques which *do not work for children from trauma*.

This tool supports an intervention which goes some way to addressing that imbalance. Armed with *The A–Z* and the BAIRT, and the tools in Parts One and Two of this book, supporting practitioners now have a strong chance of helping families to stay together and achieve positive outcomes for children.

THE BAIRT – EXAMPLE

This section contains the entire process of completing a BAIRT alongside the narrative for Josh. Later in this part, each section of the BAIRT is explained in greater detail.

DEVELOPMENTAL TRAUMA: THE BEHAVIOUR – ASSESSMENT OF IMPACT AND RESOLUTION TOOL (BAIRT) – JOSH

This assessment tool relies on the assessing supporter and therapeutic parent having access to Sarah Naish (2018) *The A–Z of Therapeutic Parenting: Strategies and Solutions.* London and Philadelphia, PA: Jessica Kingsley Publishers.

Josh is eight years old. He has been with his therapeutic foster parent Linda for three years. Linda is a single parent. She often has her five-year-old grandchild Tom to stay. Recently, Linda has begun struggling with Josh's violent outbursts. She says that he seems to get aggressive for no reason and that these episodes 'come out of nowhere'. Linda is very tired and says she feels overwhelmed. She does not know if she can continue looking after Josh anymore, as she feels drained. She is too scared to have her grandson visiting, and this is placing additional strain on her.

On 28 February Linda tells her empathic listener, Glynis, how she is feeling and Glynis realizes there are some major 'sparks' that could lead to a family breakdown and an unplanned move for Josh. Glynis also feels that Linda is showing symptoms of compassion fatigue as she says she is unable to think strategically and appears disconnected from Josh.

Glynis alerts the supervising social worker, Emma. They discuss the current situation, and consider the risks to Josh, Linda's grandson and Linda herself. They agree that Linda may be in compassion fatigue as she has stated to Emma that she feels disconnected from Josh and fearful of him. Her empathy towards him has been eclipsed by her fear for her grandson and the sadness that she is unable to see her grandson.

Glynis and Emma decide between them that Glynis will carry out the Behaviour – Assessment of Impact and Resolution Tool (BAIRT) to enable them to have a joint, clear plan with Linda and the therapeutic team to ensure that Josh can remain with Linda, and to guarantee the safety of her grandchild. Glynis is able to start the assessment the following day, as it is felt to be sufficiently urgent to re-establish stability within the family.

Glynis and Emma agree that Linda needs to be listened to and able to fully express the level of her anxiety and stress in order to reduce her levels of compassion fatigue. For this reason, they decide that the second visit will take place within 24 hours of completing the first section. They make arrangements to catch up by phone following each visit to ensure that Emma is fully appraised of the developing situation.

As a precaution, Glynis books Linda onto a training course in de-escalation, 'Managing Violent Behaviour', so that this will be available to her following this intervention.

Table 1. Comparative scores (front sheet)

Therapeutic parent	Linda Harman	
Child	Josh Williams	
Supporter	Glynis Evans	
Date of assessment	1 March	
Date of review	16 March	
	On first assessment	**On review**
Section 1: Overall behaviour score	135/332	
***** **Section 2: The three most difficult behaviours score**	25/30	
****** **Section 2: Impact on parent score**	28/30	

Notes: * Ensure that the total possible score is also noted, i.e. 3 behaviours will be out of 30, but if only 1 behaviour is recorded, it will be out of 10.

** As above, note total possible score related to the number of behaviour impacts.

Glynis phones Linda to arrange to start the assessment. They agree on mutually convenient appointments over a two-week period, with the majority of the first appointments relatively close together. Glynis explains that the front sheet will have scores added to it as they go along, and that she will be scoring Section 1 on the first assessment when they meet the next day, once they have discussed all the behaviours.

TIME FRAME

Glynis and Linda then mutually agree a time frame to complete the BAIRT as follows.

Schedule table for this assessment

Section	Recommended timings	Date and time scheduled
Section 1	1–2 hours	1 March, 2 pm–4 pm
Section 2	2 hours	2 March, 12 pm–2 pm
Section 3	2 hours	5 March, 11 am–1 pm
Section 4	2 hours	8 March, 12 pm–2 pm
Section 5	1.5 hours	16 March, 1 pm–2.30 pm

Glynis meets Linda the following day and explains that they will now start scoring an overview of all behaviours that children from trauma may often present. This is to ensure that patterns are picked up and that they don't miss anything. They reflect that it is often the case that it's easy to concentrate on one big behaviour and miss any underlying causative factors by accident. Linda says that when Josh first came to live with her there was violence, but this had been reduced after using the Developmental Foundation Planner tool (see Part Two) and other therapeutic parenting strategies.

Glynis tells Linda that the point of this part of the assessment is to merely see what leaps out. She reminds Linda that they won't be spending very long on each behaviour but that they will definitely return to any high scoring behaviours and focus on resolving these. This reassures Linda so that she does not feel anxious when Glynis keeps moving forwards.

Linda becomes tearful and distressed while completing the scoring section. She explains that the aggression and violence levels are hard to take and she does not understand why this behaviour is happening.

Glynis becomes clearer about the impact the behaviours are having and reassures Linda that the process will help to address all these issues and that they will be completing this process together. Glynis keeps the process moving forwards.

SECTION 1: THE SCOPE OF BEHAVIOURS

Briefly discuss and score each behaviour:

0 = Not present/no issues

1 = Infrequent, minor issue

2 = Sometimes problematic

3 = Frequent, problematic

4 = Severe, causes or likely to cause big problems

Record the initial score and end score.

Table 2. Complete list of behaviours

Behaviour	Initial score	End score	Behaviour	Initial score	End score
Absconding	0		Biting	2	
Absences	0		Blocking (doorways, etc.)	2	
Aggression (threatening language, etc.)	4		Boasting	1	
Alcohol	0		Brushing teeth (resistance to)	1	
Anger	4		Charming (superficial, including fake smile)	2	
Arguing (with adult)	3		Chewing	0	
Banging	2		Choosing difficulties (unable to make a choice)	0	
Bath time difficulties	1		Competitiveness (extreme)	3	
Bedtime issues	2		Contact (difficult behaviours around)	4	
Bedwetting	1		Controlling (including bullying)	4	
Birthday and other celebrations (reaction to)	2		Cruelty to animals	1	

Damaging items	2		Over-reacting	2	
Defiance	3		Poo issues	0	
Disorganization	2		Racist or sexist etc. behaviour	0	
Drugs	0		Refusing to apologize or lack of remorse	3	
Empathy (lack of, child does not care)	2		Rejecting	3	
False allegation	3		Rudeness	3	
Fearfulness	2		Running off (e.g. in sight, localized running, spur of the moment)	0	
Friendships (difficulties with)	3		Sabotaging	2	
Head banging	1		Separation anxiety	0	
Hiding	0		School issues	1	
Hoarding (food or other items)	0		Self-harm	0	
Holiday difficulties	0		Sexualized behaviour	0	
Homework	2		Shouting and/or screaming	4	
Hygiene	1		Showering	1	
Hypervigilant	2		Sibling rivalry	4 grandchild	
Hypochondria	2		Sleep issues	1	
Immature behaviour	2		Smoking	0	
Lateness (being late)	2		Sneakiness	1	
Lying	3		Social media or phone causing issues	0	
Manic laughter	1		Spitting	2	
Meal time issues	1		Staying in bed (unwilling or unable to get up)	1	
Memory issues (forgetfulness)	1		Stealing (any items excluding food)	1	
Messy bedroom	2		Sugar addiction	2	
Moaning or whining	2		Swearing	2	
Moving slowly (lagging behind)	1		Teasing	2	
Nonsense chatter or questions	1		Throwing things	2	
Obsessive	0		Transitions (not managing change)	4	
Oversensitivity to lights, loud noises, etc.	2		Triangulation (splitting)	3	

cont.

Behaviour	Initial score	End score	Behaviour	Initial score	End score
Unable to be alone	2		Urinating	1	
Ungratefulness	2		Violent (actual physical violence)	4	
Total possible	**332**		**Additional scoring**	**0**	
Actual total	**135**			**135**	

Glynis adds up the scores of all the behaviours and writes the total into the first column in Table 1. Linda could not think of any additional behaviours other than those listed in the table. She had spoken about extreme jealousy in relation to her grandchild, so Glynis recorded this under 'sibling rivalry'.

Once the scores are recorded, Glynis looks again at all the behaviours that are marked as a '4' to see what patterns are emerging. She notes, with Linda, that, as expected, issues around violence, aggression, control and anger are scoring highest, as are 'issues around contact'. They agree that this is what they will start with in their next visit. Glynis feels she has some immediate strategies but does not offer these as she knows it is the wrong time. She does, however, offer reassurance to Linda, and reminds her of support that is available out of hours.

As Linda is familiar with the term 'compassion fatigue' and understands that she may well be in compassion fatigue, she also accepts that the first stage to help her to feel better (and to be able to help Josh) will be to talk freely about how she is feeling and explore the behaviours.

Glynis and Linda revisit the time frame and check if the timings still feel okay. They agree that it is fine and arrange to meet the following day to continue the process.

SECTION 2: IDENTIFYING KEY BEHAVIOURS AND THEIR IMPACT

Impact on parent: Listening, learning and scoring

Glynis starts the second visit on a Friday by making sure that they are unlikely to be interrupted. She checks that they have privacy and that neither of them needs to rush off. Glynis understands that this part of the process is vital in enabling Linda to be able to access her own problem-solving abilities and to enable her stress levels to reduce.

Glynis explains that in this session she will be listening carefully to Linda to ascertain the impact that Josh's behaviour has on her, and also any fears Linda has for herself, Josh or others.

Glynis gives Linda her full attention during this process. Glynis does not use a laptop or any electronic device to record information. Glynis' body language is open. Glynis encourages Linda to speak openly and honestly without judgement. As Linda speaks, she becomes distressed. Glynis offers support but does not interrupt the process. She lets Linda know that she is listening by reflective, empathic commentary – for example:

- 'That sounds really hard.'
- 'How do you feel about that?'
- 'It sounds exhausting.'

As Linda describes Josh's violent outbursts, Glynis becomes aware that there may be a link to changes in contact with Josh's birth mother. She makes a mental note to hold this in mind for later sections. She does not raise this as a possibility and does not divert Linda in her exploration of the issues.

Linda describes how Josh has targeted Tom, her grandson, by pinching, hitting and slapping him. She describes how Josh tries to trap him in corners and also taunts him by taking his toys away. Linda is unable to leave them unsupervised for any length of time. Linda expresses deep sadness about this as she says, 'They used to be lovely together.'

Linda speaks about the levels of screaming and shouting that happen. She says she finds these 'ear-splitting and intolerable'.

Linda also describes high levels of violence towards her. She tells Glynis how Josh has 'lain in wait' for her and then jumped out to kick her or try and trip her up. She shows Glynis bruises on her arms where Josh has hit her with a pot plant.

Linda expresses her puzzlement over these behaviours. She is used to being an empathic therapeutic parent and is skilled in using empathic commentary. She is sad that Josh's behaviour has suddenly deteriorated to such a degree. She speaks wistfully of the warm and positive relationship they had enjoyed until recently. This reassures Glynis that there is hope for the relationship as there is still a positive connection that Linda wishes to re-establish.

Once Linda appears to have said all she needs to, she remarks that she is feeling a bit better.

Glynis opens 'Table 3: Severity and impact' of the BAIRT and suggests they now move on to look at this together.

Glynis asks Linda to identify the three key behaviours that she has been speaking about that she would now like to focus on. She asks Linda to concentrate on those that she feels are most likely to damage their relationship and/or lead to a family breakdown or an unplanned move for Josh.

Identifying key behaviours and their impact

Glynis explains that they are going to list up to three behaviours in order that Linda speaks about them. She says that the first behaviour is normally the one that requires the most attention. Glynis explains that they do not have to have three behaviours as they can stop at one or two if needed, but they cannot go beyond three. If there is a need to look at other behaviours later, Glynis clarifies that they would use a new assessment to do so.

Table 3. Severity and impact

Behaviour	Severity or frequency	Severity of impact on parent
1 Violence to Tom (grandchild)	1 2 3 4 5 6 7 8 ⑨ 10	1 2 3 4 5 6 7 8 9 ⑩
2 Shouting and screaming	1 2 3 4 5 6 7 ⑧ 9 10	1 2 3 4 5 6 7 ⑧ 9 10
3 Violent and controlling behaviours towards Linda	1 2 3 4 5 6 7 ⑧ 9 10	1 2 3 4 5 6 7 8 9 ⑩
Totals	**25**	**28**

Linda easily identifies the main behaviours that she has been speaking about with Glynis over the last hour.

Behaviour 1: As Linda has had time to process these behaviours, she is clear that the very first issue is the violence towards Tom, her grandson. This is because she feels she can no longer have Tom in the house as she fears for his safety. She scores this at 9 for severity and frequency and 10 as impact on herself. She reiterates that it is this behaviour that causes her such distress.

Behaviour 2: At first, Linda is unable to decide which behaviour should be second. She describes very upsetting 'tantrums' around contact as well as attacks on herself. Glynis explains they will just make sure they record both behaviours. Linda then decides that 'aggression around contact' may well need a similar response to the other violence-related behaviours, so she chooses 'screaming and shouting'. She says these angry outbursts happen every time they visit Josh's birth mother for contact, but also on return for the whole of the evening, sometimes well into the night. This makes her very tired.

Behaviour 3: Violent outbursts towards Linda are scored at the same level behaviourally as the issues around 'shouting and screaming', but the impact on Linda is perceived as greater. This is because she describes a feeling of 'walking on eggshells' all the time and says she finds it very difficult to relax. Linda also speaks about the level of control in relation to this behaviour. For example, she says Josh will be very confrontational, ordering her to do something, and if she doesn't comply, Josh will launch an attack. Linda says she knows she must be the 'unassailable safe base' for him, and this has repercussions for their relationship. She worries that Josh feels unsafe too.

Glynis reassures Linda that they now have some good clarity on the extent of the most pressing issues they need to deal with, and although she has some ideas and strategies, she will think about these to share next time, or in Section 4, whichever is the most appropriate. Linda says she feels better that Glynis has some ideas and does not seem fazed by the scale of the task they face. Glynis totals up the scores of the severity of the behaviours and then the impact. She adds them to Table 1, in order that they can make a comparison at the end of the process.

Glynis is aware that there must be a break between Sections 2 and 3 to enable both Linda and herself time to reflect, and to check they are not missing anything. Linda says she is feeling quite drained but also has some sense of relief. They acknowledge that this is probably due to having 'got it all out there' and to have been able to fully express the impact that these behaviours are having on Linda and on her life. Linda reflects that it's unusual as 'everyone always talks about the child and their behaviours, but they forget about us sometimes'.

Glynis reassures Linda that this process is designed to ensure that both the child and the therapeutic parent are kept in mind. Linda says that it is very powerful to see it all written down and scored, and somehow it also makes it feel more manageable.

Glynis tells Linda that she will also take time to reflect and she may also have a chat with Emma, the supervising social worker, or the attachment therapist, Julie. They confirm arrangements to meet up after the weekend on Monday.

After leaving Linda, Glynis contacts Emma to update her on progress so far. They agree that patterns are emerging around contact and violence and arrange to speak again following the third visit on Monday. Emma confirms that she has advised Josh's social worker, Ryan, about the work that is taking place and that he is happy with the decisions being made. Emma has arranged to share the results of the assessment with Ryan in order that agreement and understanding around strategies can be in place.

SECTION 3: ANALYSING THREE BEHAVIOURS

Glynis arrives as planned on Monday at 11am. She enquires about how things have been and how Linda is feeling. She finds Linda ready to get straight down to analysing the behaviours as she says she has been giving this a great deal of thought over the weekend. Linda reflects that she has not had her grandson over the weekend and there has been no contact with Josh's birth mother, so things have been relatively calm. She does disclose, however, that 'relatively calm' has still included Josh attacking her with his bike pump when she did not help him 'quickly enough'.

Glynis explains that they will now look at each behaviour in turn, and complete the column for that behaviour. She says they have approximately 30 minutes for each behaviour, and they will then spend a further 30 minutes looking at any triggers or parallels.

Thinking about each behaviour *in turn*, Glynis and Linda complete the table below, to see if further understanding can be developed and shared.

Table 4. Analysis of behaviours

	Behaviour 1: Violence to Tom (grandchild)	Behaviour 2: Shouting and screaming	Behaviour 3: Violent and controlling behaviours towards Linda
When did it start?	2 January	Early January, or possibly just after Christmas – not sure of exact date He has often screamed, but this is a new level	First week in January
Was there an obvious trigger? (Think about dates, anniversaries and changes.) If 'yes', what was the trigger?	Christmas and New Year meant Josh was out of his routine and the new school term was approaching The social worker had arranged for contact to be re-established with the birth mum and this had happened between Christmas and New Year, 28 December	Definitely when contact re-established The days leading up to 28 December were fine, but immediately following there was a very marked deterioration	After second contact on 2 January, when Linda took Josh to see his birth mum She had been advised not to say they were going for contact

	Behaviour 1: Violence to Tom (grandchild)	Behaviour 2: Shouting and screaming	Behaviour 3: Violent and controlling behaviours towards Linda
What might the child be communicating through this behaviour?	Jealousy of Tom? Anger about Linda's attention on him?	Perhaps he doesn't want to go? Maybe he is confused or frightened? Perhaps he feels torn or disloyal? Perhaps he doesn't want to return to Linda's care? Maybe he is trying not to hear what people are saying?	He feels unsafe with Linda? Perhaps he does not trust her? Is he very angry with her for something? Perhaps he is resisting a stronger attachment and trying to force a move?
Can we identify an unmet need through this behaviour?	Josh would not have had one-to-one nurturing attention when he was Tom's age. He may have been ignored, and when Linda's attention is on Tom, Josh might feel invisible, which would be frightening for him	Maybe he had many unmet needs from early-life neglect, including not being attended to when screaming?	If this is a fear-based behaviour, he might be showing us he has to be powerful and in control and is unable to allow adults to be in charge or trusted?
At what age would we normally expect to see this behaviour?	About the age of two	Not sure, but the types of tantrum and sustained screaming looks like a 'terrible twos' tantrum	Linda has seen this in younger children and also teenagers, but the type of unrealistic expectations he has, ordering her around, remind her of a young child, perhaps age two or three?
How does the parent normally respond?	Linda removes Josh from Tom and tells him he cannot play with Tom if he cannot be kind	Linda usually removes herself or puts earplugs in. She has tried other things too, like talking quietly, but this doesn't work	Linda tells Josh his behaviour is unacceptable and removes herself from his reach. Later, if injured, Linda may use logical consequences to try to make a link
How might this behaviour link back to early-life experiences? (e.g. a child shouting in bed may have been left alone in a cot)	Lack of nurture in early life. He might be 'fighting for survival' and afraid that he has been forgotten about?	Perhaps he is trying to be 'bigger' or 'angrier' or more powerful, trying to make others respond to the screaming? He would have been left alone for long periods when he was little and ignored	The need to be in control, to control adults who he believes to be unsafe? In his early life there were very few boundaries and he witnessed a lot of violence too

What strategies have already been tried?	Removing Tom from Josh Removing toys that are being used as weapons Stopping Tom visiting Increased levels of supervision Telling Josh his behaviour is unacceptable Sending Josh to his room	Preparing Josh for contact to try to keep his cortisol levels low. Also arranging calming activities afterwards, such as water play Also tried taking him to his contact with no preparation, but this made the aftermath much worse	Using logical consequences to link cause and effect, e.g. 'My arm is hurting so I can't drive' Using a strong voice, e.g. 'Stop it now'
What happened?	When removed from Tom, Josh escalated and trashed his room Josh accused Linda of 'hating him' and only 'loving Tom' Josh deliberately broke items he knew were special to Linda	First time 28 December – lots of anger and shouting before and after contact and in the intervening days Second time 2 January – prolonged screaming for 6 hours. Josh was exhausted	The logical consequences did not seem to work as he did not care, but then he got more angry about Linda not driving him to Youth Club when they had to walk. This meant they missed Youth Club as it was too difficult to manage him to get there

Parallels and triggers

Can the therapeutic parent think of any parallels from their own childhood or adult emotional experiences that make this particular behaviour especially hard to deal with? If yes, make brief notes as per the example below.

> **Notes:**
> Linda feels that a line is crossed when a child hits a parent. Her own parents were very strong on this. She also feels triggered when Josh is so unkind to Tom as she very much wants them to 'be friends' as Josh often functions at a similar emotional age. She worries that she is overreacting to this too.

After completing the analysis of the behaviours, Linda is reflective about the emotional age at which Josh appears to be functioning. It also becomes startlingly clear that all the violence-related behaviours stem from the re-introduction of contact, but that they deteriorated rapidly around the second visit. Glynis and Linda refer back to the completed Trauma Tracker for Josh for more guidance with this (see Part One).

Glynis and Linda discuss this further and speculate about the differences in how each contact visit was managed. Linda discloses that she was very uncomfortable when Josh's social worker told her that she needed to take Josh to the second contact visit without any preparation. Linda states, 'I am supposed to be his "unassailable safe base", yet I am tricking him. Well that is what it felt like in any case.' She describes Josh's reaction when he saw his birth mother just outside the family centre as 'extreme' as he was furious and tried to hide in the footwell of the car and he 'screamed for hours' afterwards.

Psycho-sensory therapy session

As clear triggers have been identified, Glynis and Linda discuss the best way to minimize or remove these triggers. Linda is familiar with psycho-sensory therapies such as mindfulness and Delta Wave Therapy (e.g. Havening Techniques®) as she has benefited from these in the past. She is open to having a Delta Wave Therapy session around removing the high emotional response she feels about Tom and also her response to Josh's screaming noises. Linda says it makes her feel as if 'her brain is shaking'. Glynis makes arrangements to refer Linda for that to happen before the next visit when they meet to discuss strategies.

The following day, Linda has a session of Delta Wave Therapeutic Touch with a practitioner, and this results in her feeling less overwhelmed and emotional when she recalls Josh targeting Tom.

SECTION 4: STRATEGIES AND SOLUTIONS

Pooling strategies

Glynis arrives as planned for Section 4. She brings with her a copy of *The A–Z* so that they can refer to this when needed for ideas. Linda updates Glynis about her Delta Wave Therapy session and says she is feeling calmer and is looking forward to exploring strategies. Glynis and Linda start by looking at Behaviour 1, and work through each behaviour in turn.

Table 5. Strategies and solutions

Behaviour 1: Violence to Tom (grandchild) – we have looked mainly at 'sibling rivalry' for indicators on this
Why might the child be doing what he or she is doing?
• Fear of invisibility, in particular the need for Linda to notice Josh above Tom, especially when the other children might be getting attention for positive *or* negative behaviours • Josh needs to feel powerful and in control • Rewards Josh with a reaction (trigger for Linda responding to the rivalry, e.g. refereeing)
Strategies we will use
• Minimize or remove physical barriers that prevent supervision – Linda will stay present or have a friend present too if Tom is visiting • Use 'showing sorry' to help Josh put things right • Create a secret 'signal' to reassure Josh that Linda is thinking of him • Linda will respond calmly without appearing angry or emotional, with empathic commentary
The best time to use these strategies
• Planning to have a friend present needs to happen prior • 'Showing sorry' needs to happen immediately following an incident, or as close as possible to the incident • Linda needs to give Josh the 'secret signal' prior to Tom visiting • Linda needs to demonstrate 'calmness' throughout a visit from Tom and prior

What might make this difficult to do? (Obstacles)

- Linda's friend may not be able to help
- Josh may be too dysregulated to engage in 'showing sorry'
- Linda may show anger and be triggered

What can we put in place to overcome these obstacles?

- The fostering agency could provide a support worker for the first visit with Tom
- 'Showing sorry' can be delayed if needed
- Linda can remove herself to calm if another person is present for Josh

Behaviour 2: Shouting and screaming

Why might the child be doing what he or she is doing?

- Fear response, especially if he feels cornered
- Fear of invisibility or of being forgotten – seeking a response, reminding others of their presence
- Fear or fearful anticipation of negative response from Linda and/or birth mum – shouting and screaming may block out a response
- Fear response of a new situation – relating to contact and also transitions with Tom visiting and routine changes re. Christmas
- Dysregulation – 'acting in the heat of the moment'. Possible sensory overload? Josh is unable to regulate or calm himself

Strategies we will use

- Think more about when Josh screams and relationship to contact and Linda's unavailability
- Parental presence to regulate with calming sounds such as low humming, quiet music, etc.
- Distraction with random statement, e.g. looking past Josh as if heard something else
- If possible, going out into the garden to take some deep breaths to regulate self
- 'Name the need' behind the shouting – Josh may be unaware that this seems to relate to contact and Linda being busy

The best time to use these strategies

- 'Naming the need' should be done when Josh is calm
- Distraction can be used in the early stages of screaming
- Will need parental presence while he is screaming
- Going out into garden will be during the incident, so care will need to be taken re. safety, etc.

What might make this difficult to do? (Obstacles)

- Linda needs some advice and help around 'naming the need'
- Linda may find it difficult to stay present and feel calm while Josh is screaming
- May be too difficult to go out into garden during an incident unless someone else is there. Worried about Josh feeling abandoned

What can we put in place to overcome these obstacles?

- Glynis and Linda will make a plan and rehearse discussions around 'naming the need' today
- Linda could listen to music on earphones, and also access additional Delta Wave Therapy to remove triggers if required
- Linda could say she needs the loo instead and go there for some deep breathing

Behaviour 3: Violent and controlling behaviours towards Linda

Why might the child be doing what he or she is doing?

- The need to be in control – Josh may be aggressive in order to gain control after feeling out of control or tricked by Linda
- Feelings of hostility or momentary hatred towards Linda or birth mum?
- A desire to break a forming attachment (with Linda)
- Sensory issues – perhaps Josh is overloaded with sensory information, during transitions?

cont.

Strategies we will use

- 'Naming the need' – Linda needs to explain to Josh that she believes he is angry with her because she took him to contact without telling him where they were going. Even though she was acting on instruction, Josh needs to hear why he is so angry with Linda and feeling unsafe, as it is likely he does not realize this
- Glynis has requested a place for Linda at 'Managing Violent Behaviour' training around de-escalation and safe holding
- Linda will start using the phrase 'I know you have a good heart'
- Linda will read *William Wobbly and the Very Bad Day* (Naish and Jefferies 2016) to help Josh realize he is not the only child experiencing this
- Linda will relate empathic commentary to what she thinks Josh is angry about, e.g. 'I am sorry you are feeling so angry with me for talking to Tom. I have not forgotten you'

The best time to use these strategies

All strategies need to happen outside of the incident, apart from empathic commentary and saying 'I know you have a good heart', which is best used at the beginning of an incident or afterwards. Linda will 'name the need' with Josh as soon as possible at the appropriate time as she feels this is key

What might make this difficult to do? (Obstacles)

No real barriers except if Josh does not engage in the *William Wobbly* story, or he may be angry and try not to hear the 'naming the need' conversation

What can we put in place to overcome these obstacles?

If Josh does not want to engage with the story, Linda will leave the book near him, or make sure Josh hears her reading it elsewhere. Linda is not concerned if Josh acts as though he cannot hear the message when she 'names the need' as she feels his behaviour afterwards will indicate whether or not he has

As Glynis and Linda work through the behaviours, in turn it becomes very obvious about the level of fear Josh is experiencing.

They discuss the possibility of this being linked to the re-introduction of contact, especially where Linda took him to the Family Centre unprepared. Linda is clear that this definitely made a big impact on Josh and triggered a lot of the violent behaviours towards her. She can see how Josh would target her if he felt she was not keeping him safe. On top of this, it appears as though Josh is more threatened by Tom being around as this may be making him feel 'invisible'.

Glynis and Linda discuss the possibility that Josh may be thinking that he is going to be rejected and returned to his birth mum (which he does not want) or moved to another foster parent. They feel that some of his behaviours are designed to break the forming attachment between Linda and Josh, which had strengthened before and around Christmas.

Linda says she now feels 'terrible' about taking Josh to contact unprepared, and can't believe that she had not properly made this link. Glynis reassures Linda that she was acting on professional advice and thought she was acting in Josh's best interests.

Glynis and Linda make practical arrangements about who will be present to support Linda and who will arrange this. Glynis tells Linda that she has managed to move her training forward for the de-escalation part of training in 'Managing Violent Behaviour', and lets her know the date.

Plan to review

Glynis and Linda decide to meet as arranged on 16 March to give Linda time to see how the strategies are working. Glynis says she will phone Linda in two days as well to see how things are going and to tweak the strategies if needed.

| The supporter will contact the parent by phone on 13 March at 2 pm to check on progress |
| We will meet to review how well this plan is going on 16 March at 1 pm |

In the meantime, the therapeutic parent will also communicate to the supporter any positive or negative changes noted in the child's behaviour.

> **Notes:**
> Linda will prioritize 'naming the need' to see if this makes an immediate impact on the severity and frequency of the behaviours. Both parties agree that it seems as if Josh has become fearful of being invisible and also has lost confidence in Linda as his 'unassailable safe base' due to the way in which the contact in early January was managed. Glynis will discuss this with the supervising social worker and Josh's social worker to ensure the ramifications of this advice are understood and not repeated.

Glynis contacts Linda, as arranged, and they discuss how things are going. Linda says she has used 'naming the need'. She says she sat down with Josh and said, 'I am so sorry that you have been feeling so wobbly. I think I made you feel wobbly because the day I took you to go and see your mum at the Family Centre, I didn't tell you she was going to be there. This was a mistake and I know that it probably made the little part of Josh feel that he couldn't trust me anymore. I promise you that I will never do that again and my job is to keep you safe.'

Linda says that although Josh seemed thoughtful and reflective, he did not say anything. She reports that since this conversation the violence has decreased markedly.

SECTION 5: REFLECTION AND REVIEW

Revisiting and rescoring

Glynis visits Linda for the final section to review how things are going. Linda describes how using 'parental presence' during Josh's tantrums where he is screaming and shouting was very difficult at first, but over the last few days this has seemed to regulate him and the screaming has decreased.

Linda also describes how the violence has decreased markedly since she did 'naming the need' around her guess that Josh had been made to feel unsafe by her. She has noticed more warmth in their relationship, although Josh is still wary. The violence against her has now virtually disappeared.

Glynis updates Linda and tells her that Emma, the supervising social worker, has been in contact with Josh's social worker and they have agreed that contact will always be spoken about openly in the future. Furthermore, they have agreed that a member of staff will take Josh to contact when it re-starts. This will mean that Linda is not in a position where she is taking Josh to the source of his fear, which is what has appeared to happen in the past, from Josh's perspective.

Glynis asks how things are with Tom and if he has visited. Linda says that they have done one short visit in a neutral location and she took a helper with her, as planned. She made sure that she had given Josh his secret signal beforehand and that seemed to work really well. For instance, when she needed to clean Tom up because he was grubby, she gave Josh a wink with a thumbs up and he was able to calm himself. Linda describes feeling on tenterhooks throughout the visit but, in fact, it went surprisingly well. She is going to try this again next week.

The strategy that was discussed around Linda removing herself in order to feel calm has not yet been used. Linda has not felt the need to do this and is feeling in control and generally much safer with Josh.

Glynis then says they need to go through all the behaviours in Table 2 and mark them again to see what changes have happened. She explains that it's important to check that some other behaviours haven't perhaps started to become more problematic, so this is why they are going to look at the whole range of behaviours again.

Table 2 revisited. Complete list of behaviours

Behaviour	Initial score	End score	Behaviour	Initial score	End score
Absconding	0	0	Controlling (including bullying)	4	2
Absences	0	0	Cruelty to animals	1	0
Aggression (threatening language, etc.)	4	2	Damaging items	2	1
Alcohol	0	0	Defiance	3	1
Anger	4	1	Disorganization	2	2
Arguing (with adult)	3	1	Drugs	0	0
Banging	2	1	Empathy (lack of, child does not care)	2	2
Bath time difficulties	1	1	False allegation	3	1
Bedtime issues	2	1	Fearfulness	2	1
Bedwetting	1	1	Friendships (difficulties with)	3	3
Birthday and other celebrations (reaction to)	2	2	Head banging	1	1
Biting	2	0	Hiding	0	0
Blocking (doorways, etc.)	2	1	Hoarding (food or other items)	0	0
Boasting	1	1	Holiday difficulties	0	0
Brushing teeth (resistance to)	1	0	Homework	2	2
Charming (superficial, including fake smile)	2		Hygiene	1	1
Chewing	0	0	Hypervigilant	2	2
Choosing difficulties (unable to make a choice)	0	0	Hypochondria	2	2
Competitiveness (extreme)	3	1	Immature behaviour	2	2
Contact (difficult behaviours around)	4	1	Lateness (being late)	2	2

Lying	3	2	Sexualized behaviour	0	0
Manic laughter	1	1	Shouting and/or screaming	4	1
Meal time issues	1	0	Showering	1	1
Memory issues (forgetfulness)	1	1	Sibling rivalry	4	1
Messy bedroom	2	2	Sleep issues	1	1
Moaning or whining	2	1	Smoking	0	0
Moving slowly (lagging behind)	1	1	Sneakiness	1	1
Nonsense chatter or questions	1	1	Social media or phone causing issues	0	0
Obsessive	0	0	Spitting	2	0
Over reacting	2	1	Staying in bed (unwilling or unable to get up)	1	1
Oversensitivity to lights, loud noises, etc.	2	2	Stealing (any items excluding food)	1	1
Poo issues	0	0	Sugar addiction	2	2
Racist or sexist etc. behaviour	0	0	Swearing	2	1
Refusing to apologize or lack of remorse	3	2	Teasing	2	1
Rejecting	3	1	Throwing things	2	0
Rudeness	3	1	Transitions (not managing change)	4	1
Running off (e.g. in sight, localized running, spur of the moment)	0	0	Triangulation (splitting)	3	2
Sabotaging	2	2	Unable to be alone	2	1
School issues	1	1	Ungratefulness	2	2
Separation anxiety	0	0	Urinating	1	0
Self-harm	0	0	Violent (actual physical violence)	4	1
Total possible	**332/332**		**Additional scoring**	**0 0**	
Actual total	**135/79**			**135/79**	

When the scoring is completed, Linda is pleased to see that the score has halved. She says, 'That's what it feels like. It isn't as if everything is magically wonderful suddenly, but it's just much more manageable.'

Glynis writes the score in Table 1, then moves on to score the three behaviours separately by using Table 6 to revisit the scores recorded in Table 3.

Looking at Table 3, recorded in Section 2, Glynis and Linda think about what has changed and score the *current* severity.

Table 6. Rescoring severity and impact

Behaviour	Severity or frequency NOW	Severity of impact on parent NOW
1 Violence to Tom (grandchild) NOW	1 2 3 ④ 5 6 7 8 9 10	1 ② 3 4 5 6 7 8 9 10
2 Shouting and screaming NOW	1 2 ③ 4 5 6 7 8 9 10	1 2 ③ 4 5 6 7 8 9 10
3 Violent and controlling behaviours towards Linda NOW	1 2 ③ 4 5 6 7 8 9 10	1 2 ③ 4 5 6 7 8 9 10
Totals	**10**	**8**

When completing Table 6, on 'Behaviour 1: Violence to Tom' Linda remarks that this is not fully tested yet as they have only had one visit. Glynis then revisits Table 1, and inserts all the scores. They can see that there is a big improvement and no other difficult behaviours seem to have arisen so far.

Table 1 revisited. Comparative scores

Therapeutic parent	Linda Harman	
Child	Josh Williams	
Supporter	Glynis Evans	
Date of assessment	1 March	
Date of review	16 March	
	On first assessment	**On review**
Section 1: Overall behaviour score	135/332	79/332
* **Section 2: The three most difficult behaviours score**	25/30	10/30
** **Section 2: Impact on parent score**	28/30	8/30

Notes: * Ensure that the total possible score is also noted, i.e. 3 behaviours will be out of 30, but if only 1 behaviour is recorded, it will be out of 10.

** As above, note total possible score related to the number of behaviour impacts.

Reviewing the process

Glynis suggests that it's now a good time to look back at the process and see what needs to happen now. She takes on board Linda's comment about the lack of opportunity so far to test out Josh's levels of violence to Tom, so this is something they will need to keep in mind. Glynis uses Table 7 to form the basis of their discussions.

Table 7. Review

How is the parent feeling about what has happened?

Linda is feeling quite amazed at the differences in both Josh's behaviour and also in how she is feeling in herself. She is very relieved that things feel more manageable at present, but is naturally cautious about expecting too much too quickly

What has the therapeutic parent learned about:

a) The child?
Josh had been very frightened, and his behaviours were a result of this fear. He had felt unsafe with Linda

b) Therapeutic parenting and child trauma?
The power of 'naming the need'. Linda did not think it would have such a marked effect so rapidly but it really resonated with Josh

c) The agency's practice?
Linda feels there has been good communication and support throughout the process. She has been relieved that issues that were picked up were discussed with Josh's social worker so she did not also need to try to explain them

What has changed?

Linda feels more in control and understands what is going on. Because of this, Josh is much calmer. There is no longer an upward spiral based on a need to control. Signals regarding future visits with Tom are promising

What still needs to change?

Tom will need to come and visit again in a structured way, in order to continue trying out Josh's tolerance levels. Contact needs to be reviewed to ensure that the triggering event can never happen again

What has the supporter learned about:

a) The child?
Josh has needed much more support around contact than was originally thought

b) The therapeutic parent?
Linda is able to communicate very effectively when she is struggling and is open and accepting of this process. She has an amazing ability to reflect and is so determined to get things right when many other foster parents would be giving up

c) Therapeutic parenting and child trauma?
The trigger from contact and how that impacted negatively on the 'unassailable safe base' relationship

d) The agency's practice?
The joined-up working within the TRUE model has enabled Glynis to stay focused on Linda's needs whilst the supervising social worker has been able to deal with the wider issues relating to practice and liaise more effectively with the local authority social worker

What has changed?

Linda is clearly much more able to cope with Josh and sees his behaviour as a communication now, rather than a threat. Her reflective practice has enabled Josh to become more regulated and his violent behaviours have diminished as a direct result

What still needs to change?

We need to be vigilant around Josh's interactions with Tom and make sure we can enable Linda's relationship with her grandson to continue unhindered

How will this be changed?

We may need to consider helping Josh to go for regular 'sleepovers' at a friend's house to enable Linda to have uninterrupted visits from her grandson occasionally

Signatures

	Signed	Date
Assessment concluded	*(signature)*	16/03/21
Therapeutic parent		
Therapeutic parent		
Supporter		

HOW TO USE THE BAIRT

It is a good idea to refer back to the completed BAIRT alongside the explanation in this section.

Considerations before starting the BAIRT

Before setting out on an assessment, the supporter and team around the family will have become aware of some indicators, some 'sparks'. It is essential, of course, to consider the safety of the child before starting out on the assessment. In an ideal situation the types of sparks that may be noticed will relate to a deteriorating relationship or the therapeutic parent beginning to struggle to manage the child's behaviours, or a noticeable withdrawal. Sometimes there may be a need for the child to move to a short break family while work is carried out with the parents. Obviously, the safety of the child is paramount, but it is also important to balance the needs of the child and the child's perspective with the reality of the situation. If it is felt that the family can be stabilized quite quickly through the use of this tool and there is no risk to the child, then clearly the child should remain within the family.

The BAIRT can be used in order to help the child stay in the family, and significant improvements should be noted in relationships within the first two visits of the intervention.

Where the stress levels of the therapeutic parent are thought to be exceptionally high, the supporter should plan to complete Sections 1 and 2 within the same visit. This will enable the supporter to offer active empathic listening throughout the visit to help reduce the therapeutic parent's stress levels more quickly.

Midway through the assessment, the supporter may need to refer the parent for an intervention to remove triggers using psycho-sensory-integrated therapies such as mindfulness, relaxation therapies, guided meditation, Delta Wave Therapy, EMDR (Eye Movement Desensitization and Reprocessing), etc. The supporter should have a good understanding of what is available locally, and ensure this can be in place where needed.

Where clearly identified problems relating to 'child-to-parent violence' are reported, the BAIRT should not be seen as an alternative to putting in place the correct level of face-to-face training, such as 'Managing Violent Behaviour', where necessary. It is a good idea to identify and book the necessary training alongside carrying out the BAIRT, and this should be planned at an early stage.

Identifying the supporter (assessor)

The person who is going to carry out the assessment should be referred to as the 'supporter'. Ideally it will be someone who knows the family well. Thought will need to be given to who is the best person to carry out the assessment and intervention. The supporter needs to be aware that the parent will be feeling vulnerable and anxious and unlikely to want to embark on a new relationship. Ideally the person who is best placed to carry out the assessment and intervention will be someone who is trusted by the parent and in an established relationship with them.

Due to the construction of the assessment tool, however, it is possible to introduce a new person just for the work to be carried out. It must be stressed that this is far from ideal, and extra visits may need to be bolted on to the beginning of the intervention to ensure a basis of trust is established.

Within the TRUE model (explained in the 'Introduction' to this book) I have clarified that we would normally have an empathic listener who is introduced to the family at a very early stage. It is always useful that the person who is carrying out the assessment is someone who knows what the family is like normally as well as during a crisis too.

The supporter must remain consistent throughout the assessment and must not hand over to another supporting professional midway through.

It is therefore essential to ensure that time is available to complete this assessment, and to prioritize this time.

The supporter must put aside the time for the assessment and commit to it. This is to ensure that the therapeutic parent does not have to repeat themselves or lose trust in the supporting professionals during a critical process.

Where a supporter fails to engage and adhere to the agreed timescales, this sends a powerful message to the therapeutic parent. The message is received as 'I am not worth your time. My priorities are not your priorities.'

For a parent struggling with day-to-day difficulties and intense behaviours, something that appears as simple as a missed appointment can be the catalyst for an unplanned move and family breakdown.

Engaging the parent

It's important to remember that where parents are in compassion fatigue, they are very likely to view the introduction of an assessment tool negatively. At these times when parents are struggling, everything can feel overwhelming and like 'yet another task', or worse, a form of criticism or blame. It is therefore essential (and perfectly possible) to introduce the tool in such a way that does not feel onerous. For example, a supporter can be empathic on a phone call and say:

> I can see things are feeling really difficult at the moment. I'm going to come round to visit you to see what I can do to help.

In this way the first visit of the assessment can easily be done as a fact find, and the rest of the process follows naturally on from there. Although it's advisable to share with the parent that this is a process the supporting professionals and parent are starting and will be completing together, where the parent is overwhelmed there is no harm in approaching this in a bite-size manner, rather than turning up with pages of documents that need to be completed! This will likely disengage the parent at an early stage.

I would always recommend that a supporter planning to visit a parent who is exhausted and stressed goes to visit with a lovely nurturing gift. This might be chocolate, cake, a bath bomb or even some nice coffee. The importance of this message should not be underestimated. After all, how often do we visit therapeutic parents and accept *their* hospitality? A nurturing gift says to the therapeutic parent, 'I was thinking of you. I know you are struggling. I care. I want to help you feel better.' It also gives the parent the important message that they are not alone.

Setting the scene

In an ideal situation the parent and supporter will already be familiar with the BAIRT. This may have been covered during the assessment of foster parents or adopters, for example, or during early training. It's a good idea to introduce familiarity with the tool at an early stage so that the parent does not feel that this is an unfamiliar and worrying development being introduced at a time when they are already suffering increased levels of stress.

If the terminology around 'sparks' has previously become mainstream in conversations with parents, it's an easy leap for supporting professionals to introduce the idea of bringing in the assessment tool to help the parent with constructive, meaningful support. For example:

> I've noticed a few 'sparks' recently where you've raised issues around Josh's behaviour. Have you noticed them too?

This type of language avoids blame and starts from a point of curiosity.

Therapeutic parents are used to having assessments and, of course, adopters and foster parents have been through comprehensive assessment processes. Sometimes the need for an assessment is not viewed positively by those caring for children from trauma. This is due to the fact that assessment often leads to no action, or worse, blame. Many parents will have experienced multiple assessments that led to no action or improvements. We are all familiar with scenarios where meetings are called, assessments carried out, but then recommendations fail to be acted on.

Therefore, assurances need to be given at an early stage, that the point of the assessment tool is to lessen the impact on the parents and to help find strategies to resolve the situation. Emphasize that this will be carried out with just the supporter and therapeutic parent together. They will be in charge, jointly, of the timescales and outcomes for the assessment.

This ensures that the parent *feels* empowered, *is* empowered and takes an active part in the process. So the parent moves from the feeling that they are 'being assessed' (yet again) towards active assistance in finding resolutions.

Outline of the sections

The BAIRT consists of five sections that are worked through together by the supporter and parent together:

Section 1: The scope of behaviours. This enables the supporter and therapeutic parent to work together to establish a comprehensive overview of any presenting behaviours that may be causing the issues.

Section 2: Identifying key behaviours and their impact on the parent. In this section the supporter uses empathic listening to allow the therapeutic parent the time and space to properly discuss and identify the most difficult behaviours, enabling them to feel heard without blame or judgement.

Section 3: Analysing three behaviours. This section identifies up to three key behaviours and looks more deeply into each behaviour, analysing where the behaviour might stem from.

Section 4: Strategies and solutions. This section relies on the supporter and therapeutic parent using their pooled knowledge, alongside *The A–Z*, to look at which strategies might work best with the child, what might make this difficult, and when is the best time to start using them.

Section 5: Review and reflection. In this section the supporter and therapeutic parent assess the effectiveness of the intervention so far, and plan any further changes or support needed.

List of tables

Table name	Position and purpose
Schedule table for assessment	Front sheet, used prior to visit 1 and amended or updated in visit 1
	Timetable agreement for planning dates and times
Table name	**Position and purpose**
Table 1. Comparative scores	Front sheet, used in visits 1 and 5
	Captures scores at the beginning and end of the process for quick comparison
Table 2. Complete list of behaviours	Section 1, used in visit 1 and revisited in visit 5
	Complete list of behaviours from *The A–Z* for reference, discussion and scoring
Table 3. Severity and impact	Section 2, used in visit 2 and compared with updated version (Table 6) in visit 5
	Measures initial scores (0–10 severity) of up to three behaviours, and also the severity of the impact of these behaviours on the therapeutic parent
Table 4. Analysis of behaviours	Section 3, used in visit 3
	An overview of each behaviour in comparison format, to identify what has been tried, effectiveness, triggers, patterns and parallels

cont.

Table 5. Strategies and solutions	Section 4, used in visit 4
	Three identical tables to look at each behaviour one at a time in detail, to identify what is being communicated by the child and to agree on appropriate strategies
Table 6. Rescoring severity and impact	Section 5, used in visit 5
	Revisiting Table 3 for comparative scoring. Identical to Table 3, except it is updated in review
Table 7. Review	Section 5, used in visit 5
	A review of the intervention, effectiveness and any further actions required

Time frame

The assessment will usually be carried out with a supporter, over five to six visits with the therapeutic parent.

Where there is a current crisis, the supporter will need to complete Sections 1 and 2 on the same day and then arrange to start Section 3 within 24 hours. There must be a gap of at least 24 hours between Sections 2 and 3 to allow the therapeutic parent time to recover.

Where the issue is of a less urgent nature, it is possible to do weekly visits, covering one section per week.

It goes without saying that the therapeutic parent must also prioritize the assessment as a way to resolve current difficulties.

Each family will be different, requiring more or less time with their supporter.

The initial appointment will usually be made by email or by phone. If it is felt appropriate, and the parent is engaged, the remainder of the schedule table can be completed prior to the first visit.

Visit 1: planning and information gathering

If a supporter has arrived into a very highly charged situation, it is perfectly possible to merge Sections 1 and 2, if these are carried out within the same visit. For example, it might be the case that when the supporter arrives, the therapeutic parent is so distressed or angry that they are unable to focus on starting the assessment. Empathic listening will need to happen before any work can be started. Once the therapeutic parent is calmer, the supporter can guide back towards the tables that need completing.

It is likely that a supporter will arrive in a situation where the parent is feeling overwhelmed. This may be communicated through:

- Anger.
- Blaming the fostering agency or worker.
- Exhaustion.
- Blaming the child.
- Negativity towards the child.
- Ultimatums.

- Sadness or distress.
- Withdrawal.
- Despondency.
- Catastrophic thinking.
- Defensiveness.
- Attempting to reassure the supporter that all is well.

It will be necessary to give assurances that this process is designed to work through the issues step by step, to help the family come to a resolution.

Where the supporter is met with high levels of emotion, they must put to one side any documents and *listen*. There will be a need to allow the therapeutic parent to be able to regulate themselves by expressing their stress. This is the most effective way of being able to move on. The supporter must reassure the parent that the whole process relies on them, as a supporter, getting a deep understanding of the situation they are dealing with, and the impact this is having on the parent.

As Section 2 will use empathic listening to help to reduce stress levels, a skilled supporter will be able to merge Sections 1 and 2 to use empathic listening throughout, as required.

If the schedule table has not been completed prior, a good neutral way of starting is by timetabling in appointments.

When appropriate, the therapeutic parent and supporter should complete the table below together to help to plan the assessment. As a *minimum*, each assessment should allow the times specified in the second column, but this can be increased as required. It is recommended that extra time is allocated in the diaries of both parties in case the appointment runs over.

Schedule table for assessment: timetable for planning

Section	Recommended timings	Date and time scheduled
1	1–2 hours	
2	2 hours	
3	2 hours	
4	2 hours	
5	1.5 hours	

FRONT SHEET: INITIAL SCORING (TABLE 1)

Although Table 1 appears on the front sheet (for ease of reference), it is completed at the *end* of Section 1, once the scope of the behaviours has been discussed and scored. The table is then revisited for updated scores to be added for comparison, following completion of the final review section.

This allows the supporter and therapeutic parent to record scores of the impact and severity of the behaviours and easily compare scores from the beginning and end of the assessment. This scoring is an essential part of the process as it enables all parties to gauge quickly what improvements have been made and how outcomes have been changed. It is also particularly useful for fostering and adoption teams who need to gather evidence for care inspections from Ofsted and Care Inspectorate Wales (CIW).

Table 1. Comparative scores

	On initial assessment	On review
Section 1: Overall behaviour score	Insert initial total from Table 2	Insert review total from Table 2
* Section 2: The three most difficult behaviours score (reviewed and updated in Section 5)	Insert initial total from Table 3	Insert review total from Table 6
** Section 2: Impact on parent score (reviewed and updated in Section 5)	Insert total from Table 3	Insert review total from Table 6

Notes: * Ensure that the total possible score is also noted, i.e., 3 behaviours will be out of 30, but if only 1 behaviour is recorded it will be out of 10.

** As above, note total possible score related to the number of behaviour impacts.

COMPLETION OF SECTION 1

In this section the supporter uses Table 2 to score all of the behaviours listed from *The A–Z*. As there are over 60 different behaviours, it's important not to spend too long on each behaviour. This section merely allows both parties to start to highlight the areas that the assessment will need to concentrate on. Patterns will begin to emerge during this section.

A skilled supporter will quickly see the types of behaviour that cross over and link. For example, a parent may be struggling with the child's control issues and also experience that as defiance.

The behaviours are briefly discussed and then scored from 0 to 4:

- 0 = Not present/no issues
- 1 = Infrequent, minor issue
- 2 = Sometimes problematic
- 3 = Frequent, problematic
- 4 = Severe, causes/likely to cause big problems.

It can be tempting for the supporter to get side-tracked during this section and start problem-solving. This temptation *must* be resisted as it will derail the entire process.

There is no 'good' or 'bad' score as these will be subjective dependent on the therapeutic parent's frame of mind and current experience. The aim of scoring the entire range of behaviours is to gain an overview of which behaviours the parent speaks about the most and becomes 'stuck' on. This gives a good indicator of the areas to focus on.

It is possible that a parent may present a behaviour that does not seem to be covered. If the supporter has a copy of *The A–Z* with them, they can look up any topics and see which behaviour they are cross-referenced to. For example, a parent might be looking to score 'anger' but in *The A–Z* this is separated out more specifically and addressed under 'Aggression', 'Arguing' and 'Rudeness'. It's a good idea to try and be specific about the presenting behaviours as far as possible.

It would be very unlikely to find that the presenting behaviour is not listed at all in relation to other topics, but in case the parent feels they would like to keep a specific description, this can be added and scored separately on the table.

Once the scores have been totalled up, the total scores from this section must then be added to Table 1 in Section 1 in the 'On initial assessment' section.

If it has been decided that Section 2 will take place separately, then at the end of the session, the supporter must reassure the therapeutic parent that they will be thinking about the issues that have been raised. If it is planned to discuss these behaviours with other supporting professionals, tell the parent whom you will be discussing this with, and why.

Visit 2: listening and supporting

This visit needs to take place in an environment where the therapeutic parent feels they can speak freely and openly. It would not be appropriate to carry out empathic listening in an office environment. As mentioned, sometimes, if time allows and it feels right, this section may flow naturally from, or merge with, Section 1.

In Section 2 it is crucial to start to alleviate the effects of compassion fatigue. It is very likely that the therapeutic parent will be in compassion fatigue. This means they are unable, or limited in their ability:

- To hear strategies and solutions.
- To implement strategies.
- To access empathy.

Compassion fatigue comprises two separate but related dimensions: burnout and secondary traumatic stress. Burnout measures some of the negative effects of being in a helping profession and is also associated with an unsupportive work environment. It is characterized by feeling hopeless, inadequate, disconnected and overwhelmed.

No one told us it would be like this. (Ottaway and Selwyn 2016)

When a parent is in compassion fatigue real physiological changes take place in the brain. Often, a parent of a traumatized child might be judged as if this was a purely emotional response (accusations of 'coldness' and 'scapegoating' are commonplace), but the brain is, in fact, taking action to safeguard the wellbeing of the parent. Some practitioners refer to this as 'blocked care', and it is true that there does appear to be a blockage where the parent is unable to connect with the child. It must be remembered, however, that the working environment and the frustrations that are associated with it can also cause compassion fatigue.

Where the brain is blocked and the parent is in compassion fatigue, they are unable to access the prefrontal cortex, which is why their access to strategic thinking and empathy is temporarily unavailable. Active, empathic listening lowers stress levels and enables the parent to access their prefrontal cortex, often leading to a 'light bulb' moment.

The supporter must reduce the parent's stress levels through active, empathic listening without offering solutions, in order to assist them in accessing empathy for the child and to begin to formulate a strategy.

Section 2: Identifying key behaviours and their impact

LISTENING, LEARNING AND SCORING

Throughout the assessment it is necessary to resist the temptation to use a laptop or another electronic device to record information. The assessment lends itself to a paper-based format that can easily be transcribed later. There is nothing more offputting to a parent, who is trying to offload and communicate, than the back of a laptop screen with the top of someone's head tapping away on a keyboard! This removes eye contact and increases the anxiety of the therapeutic parent about how what they are saying is being interpreted.

Ensure that the parent has been given time in a safe, non-judgemental space, to fully explore and explain:

- The impact the child's behaviour has on them.
- Any fears of concerns for self, the child or others.

The supporter must ensure that the parent feels listened to and valued, and that they are not alone with these issues. It can be very difficult not to stray into discussing strategies, but this is not the right time. If the empathic listening is cut short, the therapeutic parent will feel alone and is likely to withdraw further. Strategies must not be offered at this point.

Where the supporter is working with two parents, they must be offered their own individual visit in this section, as their experiences may be very different. It is not uncommon to find that one parent, the main caregiver, suffers higher levels of intensity than the other.

HOW TO LISTEN EMPATHICALLY

Over the years I have seen many well-meaning social workers attempting to make parents feel better by saying things such as:

- 'I know exactly what you mean.'
- 'My child is just the same.'
- 'I have a teenager too; they can be difficult, can't they?'
- 'What have you done about that?'
- 'I think you need respite.'

All of these types of comments are extremely unhelpful and are likely to push parents more deeply into compassion fatigue and cause a disconnect. It is never appropriate for a supporter to compare their own situation or their own children with what the therapeutic parent is experiencing at these times. The only exception to this might be if the supporter is looking after children from trauma and has genuinely been through the same experience. During empathic listening, however, it's more appropriate to reflect on this at the end of the session, once the parent has finished speaking.

It is much more helpful to encourage the parents to continue to talk by ensuring that:

- Body language is attentive, open and honest.
- Phones are on silent and put away.

- Laptops are shut.
- Encouragement to continue is given.

Useful phrases to encourage connection might be:

- 'I am here for you.'
- 'That sounds so exhausting.'
- 'How have you been coping?'
- 'It sounds relentless.'
- 'Tell me more.'

Any attempt to make comparisons can quickly close a parent down. The physiological changes we need to happen in the brain will happen through active empathic listening. This session must not be underestimated in the importance of the whole process. I have worked with many parents where one hour of active empathic listening has enabled the parent to find their own solutions and to move on in a positive way.

If a parent is struggling to speak about the issues they are facing, then Table 3 can be introduced early on in this session to facilitate the conversation.

IDENTIFYING KEY BEHAVIOURS AND THEIR IMPACT

During the session it will become obvious which behaviours are the most likely to damage relationship building and/or lead to family breakdown. When appropriate, the supporter will use Table 3 to list up to three behaviours in order of difficulty, 1 being the most difficult (or most pressing) issue. If there is only one behaviour, then the assessment can continue to focus on just that one aspect.

Once the parent has spoken about the behaviour, the supporter must ask about the impact on the parent, if they have not already spoken about it, using questions such as:

- 'Does it affect your sleep?'
- 'Are you able to concentrate?'
- 'Are you eating okay?'

The actual score on both the severity and impact of the behaviours must be given by the parent and not the supporter. It is the therapeutic parent's perspective we are trying to take here.

Table 3. Severity and impact

Behaviour	Severity or frequency	Severity of impact on parent
1	1 2 3 4 5 6 7 8 9 10	1 2 3 4 5 6 7 8 9 10
2	1 2 3 4 5 6 7 8 9 10	1 2 3 4 5 6 7 8 9 10
3	1 2 3 4 5 6 7 8 9 10	1 2 3 4 5 6 7 8 9 10
Totals	Add up and insert in Table 1	Add up and insert in Table 1

The total scores from this section must then be added to Table 1, in the 'On initial assessment' column.

There must be a break between Sections 2 and 3 where the supporter leaves the therapeutic parent for a minimum of 4 hours, but preferably for at least 24 hours. It is likely that the therapeutic parent will start to feel better, or at least experience some relief. The break is to enable both parties to reflect. The therapeutic parent will need recovery time and the supporter will need time and space to ensure the rest of the therapeutic team are aware of progress so far. Advice may also need to be sought from the therapeutic (DDP) lead or other members of the team regarding next steps, analysis and safeguarding.

Visit 3: analysis of behaviours

It is likely that there will be some contact between the supporter and the therapeutic parent between visits 2 and 3. We would normally expect to see a clearing of the ways and some improvement in the way that the therapeutic parent is feeling. It may be that the active empathic listening has enabled the therapeutic parent to continue discussing these issues by phone between visits.

As stress levels should now be lower and there is an indication of the behaviours that the supporter and therapeutic parent need to focus on, now is the time to start really analysing these behaviours, looking at where they come from, so they can plan what they're going to do together.

Section 3: Analysing three behaviours

It is difficult to change or resolve trauma-based behaviours without recognition of *why* they occur. This section also enables the therapeutic parent to reflect on links back to early childhood trauma, and their own triggers. It is possible that a clear and identifiable trigger will emerge. Where an identified trigger is found in Section 3, it is a good idea to resolve this trigger, either through discussion or psycho-sensory therapies (such as Delta Wave Therapy, mindfulness, etc.) prior to implementing strategies. These are explained in more detail at the end of this section.

Thinking about each behaviour *in turn* (from the previous visit), the supporter completes each section in a table format with the therapeutic parent. There are three separate columns, one for each identified behaviour. This process will enable both parties to see if further understandings around *why* the behaviours are happening can be developed and shared. It is particularly useful to revisit the Trauma Tracker (see Part One of this book) at this point where one has been completed for this child.

Amending Table 4 of the BAIRT

Table 4 helps both parties to look at each behaviour in turn and to find patterns, triggers and parallels.

The supporter and therapeutic parent may need to refer to *The A–Z* for help with this section. For example, if one of the behaviours being discussed is 'difficulties with friendships', then the section on 'Friendships' in *The A–Z* suggests indicators of why a child might be behaving this way. It is very likely that one of the suggestions will resonate with the therapeutic parent.

The questions relating to each behaviour are as follows:

1. When did it start?

An approximate date or age or stage of the child is useful to record here. Also record whether this is the first time these behaviours have happened or if this has happened in several different cycles.

2. Was there an obvious trigger? (Think about the Trauma Tracker – anniversaries, dates and changes.) If 'yes', what was the trigger?

Where a Trauma Tracker has been completed, this will provide an excellent source of information around dates and triggering events. A trigger for the child is not always obvious, and may, in fact, never be found. It is too easy to make assumptions about what may be a trigger. The child's perspective is different from ours! I have known children to have been triggered by:

- Flies.
- Flushing toilets.
- Change of a parent's expression.
- Any change in routine, however slight.
- Moving from one activity to another.
- A teacher changing their glasses.
- The noise of hairdryers.

This is why it is often difficult to guess at the trigger. A useful exercise is to look at the behaviour under discussion in *The A–Z* and to see if anything resonates in the 'Why it might happen' section.

3. What might the child be communicating through this behaviour?

Again, looking at the 'Why it might happen' section on the particular behaviour within *The A–Z* will assist the supporter and therapeutic parent in identifying what the child might be communicating through the behaviour. For example, under 'sibling rivalry' one of the points is: 'A fight for survival, recreating early childhood patterns, especially where there was abuse or neglect.' Reading this, a parent may feel instinctively that the child is communicating their fear that they may be ignored and suffer as a consequence.

4. Can we identify an unmet need through this behaviour?

Question 4 is a natural extension from Question 3. Using the example above, we might feel that the unmet need, relating to this behaviour, was that the child was not kept in mind by the early-life parent. Perhaps they were ignored, isolated, scared and alone. The child needed nurture, interaction, food, warmth and safety. Some or all of this may have been absent. Some or all of that would be the unmet need, but it is useful to try to narrow it down to a few words in the description.

5. At what age would we normally expect to see this behaviour?

As discussed in Part Two of this book (the Developmental Foundation Planner), it is common for behaviours to present as ones we would normally expect to see in a much younger child. This age-inappropriateness is usually what makes the behaviours unacceptable. For example, a two-year-old screaming and shouting in a supermarket might not be seen as abnormal, but it would not be expected from an 11-year-old.

6. How does the parent normally respond?

We need to record what the normal response has been from the parent. This is different from the strategies used, addressed below. This question helps to identify triggers, which we look at later in this section. Here, we are trying to understand the emotional state of the parent when they are met with this behaviour, and how they react.

7. How might this behaviour link back to early-life experiences? (e.g. a child shouting in bed may have been left alone in a cot)

This question helps the parent and supporter to consolidate their thinking from Questions 3 and 4. *The A–Z* can be used to help to explore this under the 'Why this might happen' section relating to the particular behaviour. More often than not, the behaviours we see from children who have experienced early-life trauma are fear-based survival behaviours. This question helps to re-awaken empathy for the child.

8. What strategies have already been tried?

It is important to record what strategies have been used. If the parent is in a heightened emotional state and applying strategies half-heartedly or in a haphazard manner, they are likely to be ineffective. Now is *not* the time to add criticism or judgement around these strategies. The process allows for reflection on the effectiveness of which strategies work and which do not.

9. What happened?

In order to help to establish which strategies might be salvageable, which might need tweaking and which need eliminating, we need to record their effectiveness. It is likely that later on in this process, the parent will be able to reapply some of these strategies, but because they will be able to be more consistent and calmer in their approach, the same strategies will be more effective.

The purpose of these questions is to establish what the patterns of the behaviours are and to remind all parties about the emotional age the child may be functioning at. This allows everyone to rediscover empathy for the child and to start to view the behaviours from the child's perspective.

Within this particular process, it is essential to remind ourselves that the child is not doing this *to* us. They are just doing it. Also, the child is often unaware of the impact of their behaviours and is almost certain to be oblivious as to why they are behaving the way they are. At present, the only internal dialogue the child is likely to have is: 'I am bad, I do bad things.'

Using therapeutic parenting we *never* ask the child why they are behaving the way they are. This is unlikely to shed any light on the presenting issue and reinforces the sense of hopelessness and shame for the child. It is up to the supporter and the therapeutic parent to work out the 'why'. In this way, later on they can at least share their thoughts and suggest an explanation through 'naming the need' (see Naish 2018, p.57).

During this question-and-answer exploration, the supporter needs to be alert to renewed signs of empathy towards the child, and taking the child's perspective.

PARALLELS AND TRIGGERS

Once each behaviour has been explored in turn, it is likely that issues and thoughts will arise. The parent may have a light bulb moment, or they may feel that a particular behaviour is very triggering for them. They may offer an explanation about why this is the case. It is also possible that the parent will know they are triggered but not understand why.

In this part of the assessment, we give time, energy and thought to these matters. A supporter might guess at the reasons why the parent is triggered, but a more skilled approach is to allow the parent to discover this link for themselves. We ask the parent if they can think of any parallels from their own childhood or adult emotional experiences that make this particular behaviour especially hard to deal with. Once a trigger is identified, we can work on removing it. If it is ignored, we become locked into a circle where the behaviour continues to trigger the parent, they continue to react, and the child, rewarded by the response, continues or escalates the behaviour. Therefore, the removal of the trigger becomes an essential part of breaking the negative behaviour cycle.

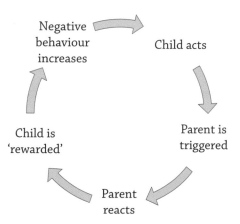

When parents are able to step back, think logically and refrain from responding emotionally, they become a very skilled therapeutic parent, with a natural 'pause' to consider challenging behaviours.

IDENTIFICATION OF TRIGGERS

Sometimes it is not easy to find an obvious link to a trigger from a difficult behaviour, but often it is clear.

Where a child is violent towards another child, for example, the trigger is obvious – fear for the other child's safety. In this type of incident we need to get the therapeutic parent to look very closely at how they respond and what the child is seeing. Some indicators for discussion around this will have presented themselves in Questions 8 and 9 above, outlining the way the parent has already responded to these behaviours, and the outcome.

Occasionally, some detective work around triggers is required. For example, a parent may say they cannot get past the fact that the child will not sit at the table and is always getting up and wandering around. Examples of hidden triggers for this might be:

- Feelings of loss of control (perhaps ask if there has been a time in their life when they felt that they had lost control of something?).
- Early childhood experience of being made to sit at a table and feeling some fear around this (note that this can be linked to the example above).
- Fear of what the child might do out of eyesight (perhaps ask if something happened to this child, or someone else, when out of eyesight? What might the child do?).

Once the triggers have been identified, sometimes they can be lowered, or removed, simply by a conscious recognition that they exist. It is a useful exercise to encourage the parent to say out loud why this trigger should be removed. For example:

> It is not Josh's fault that my dad used to make me sit at the table all afternoon. That is a separate issue and does not belong to him.

Where triggers are more entrenched and harder to overcome, we have found the use of integrated psycho-sensory techniques to be a real game-changer. The supporter can assist the therapeutic parent in accessing psycho-sensory therapies such as Delta Wave Therapy. This intervention should take place before progressing to Section 4. It will be much easier for the parent and supporter to plan effective strategies once the triggers have been recognized and removed or diminished.

THE USE OF PSYCHO-SENSORY THERAPIES (BETWEEN SECTIONS 3 AND 4)

These quick and accessible interventions are extremely useful for removing an emotional response to triggering behaviours.

Guided relaxations with meditation and mindfulness help the parent to gain a better perspective on the presenting challenges and can assist them in 'stepping' outside the moment for a different perspective.

We have found the most dramatically effective intervention of all psycho-sensory therapies are those based on Delta Wave Therapy. These include relatively new therapies such as EMDR (Eye Movement Desensitization and Reprocessing).

At the Centre of Excellence in Child Trauma,[1] we have used Delta Wave Therapy on parents who have felt they can no longer continue. This new and ground-breaking intervention is based on neuroscience. We almost always see very quick recovery as the parent re-engages with the child with renewed empathy.

At the time of publication this method is part of a joint research project with the University of Bristol to evaluate the impact of Delta Wave Therapy on parents who are in compassion fatigue.

---

1   For more information on all these psycho-sensory techniques, visit the Centre of Excellence in Child Trauma at www. coect.co.uk

Another therapy using delta waves to lower triggers and change trauma responses is the Havening Techniques. The pioneer of this method, Dr Steven Ruden, has provided this explanation:

> The Havening Techniques are a rapid, gentle and effective approach for helping people overcome anxiety based problems. Distressing feelings such as intermittent panic, stress from trauma, chronic pain, fears, depression, addictions and other related issues are amenable to Havening...the brain is an electro-chemical-magnetic organ. Pharmaceuticals address the chemical imbalance and as long as the drug is in the system its effects are present. Havening harnesses the electrical side (electroceutical), and through a simple protocol introduces delta waves into the mind/body system. Delta waves are very special in that they are normally absent during the awake hours and are primarily present during sleep when thoughts are stored. The mind/body holds memories. Sometimes these memories create symptoms and the use of an electroceutical (something that causes an effect due to an electrical wave) is able to alter those encoded ideas and remove their effect from our system. This removal changes both the underlying stressor and the individual's response.[2]

PLANNING FOR SUCCESS

Between Sections 3 and 4, the supporter should discuss the analysis of the behaviours with the team around the family, in particular the supervising social worker, empathic listener and attachment therapist (where available).

Pooled knowledge can be extremely useful in these situations, and will ensure that the supporter can return to complete Section 4, feeling confident.

Visit 4: agreeing strategies

Ideally a gap of less than seven days will take place between Sections 3 and 4, which will be just enough time to allow for any additional therapeutic intervention. Where this is not been necessary, Section 4 can be completed very soon after Section 3, even within 24 hours.

If the parent is still highly emotional and unable to look at the behaviours strategically, it may be necessary to return to empathic listening to try to identify anything that has been missed, or simply to allow the parent more time to regulate.

This is especially relevant where there has been a new incident that may need exploring and an empathic, thoughtful response. Never be worried about moving back a stage in the process. If the supporter quells anxieties and 'hopes for the best', it is likely that this approach will mean having to put in a great deal more time at a later date.

Where the therapeutic parent has accessed a psycho-sensory therapy session to address the trigger, the supporter will start the visit by checking how this went. A successful therapeutic intervention will normally lead the parent to be very positive and likely to appear in quite a different frame of mind.

The supporter and parent will naturally discuss the identified triggers and behaviours.

---

2   See www.havening.org

The supporter may notice that the parent has already started revisiting strategies and possible solutions.

Now is the time to build on the identified behaviours, implement the strategies and to then make a plan to review the application of these strategies to gauge their effectiveness.

Where the trigger for the behaviour has been successfully removed, we can start to see different outcomes ahead. If the child is met with an empathic or thoughtful response from the therapeutic parent (due to the fact that the parent is no longer triggered), the child is likely to be regulated by the parent's response and the negative behaviour will decrease. Our ideal aim is for the therapeutic parent to have stopped *reacting* and to have started *responding*.

Sometimes the simple removal of the trigger is all that is necessary to happen in order to resolve the behavioural issues and stress levels within the parent. The two often go hand in hand.

When we consider 'The PARENTS Model' (Naish 2018, pp.41–50), we know that the very first stage is 'Pause'. The parent needs to be able to pause and think reflectively in order to respond appropriately. This is why the supporter and therapeutic parent have put so much work in, before even starting to look at strategies.

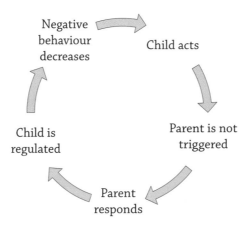

If strategies are found to fail or to be less effective than anticipated, it is also essential to revisit Section 3 to double-check that the thinking behind the cause of the behaviours is right. The supporter and parent may wish to involve the rest of the therapeutic team around the child if they feel they are not making progress at this point or if they feel the issues are too complex. In these circumstances *it is vital that the team who join these discussions are skilled and knowledgeable in child trauma and therapeutic parenting.*

MANAGING 'EEYORE PARENTS'

In *The Quick Guide to Therapeutic Parenting* (Naish and Dillon 2020) I describe a mindset that is easy to fall into for parents as 'Eeyore parenting'. I've based this on a scene from *Christopher Robin* where Eeyore is floating helplessly towards the weir and Christopher Robin is attempting to help him. Eeyore is unable to accept or recognize any help and has an extremely gloomy outlook accepting his plight.

Where a parent is struggling to accept help and is fixated on negative outcomes (and the steps around resolving compassion fatigue have been revisited to no avail), it is possible that they will naturally have a negative outlook and indulge in catastrophic thinking.

I understand that our children can overwhelm and frustrate us, and it is not unusual for a parent to experience this mindset at times. It is essential, however, that the supporter helps the parent out of this mindset. Our main tool has been empathic listening to help resolve this, but where the parent is stuck, sometimes we need some tough love.

In training, where a parent has been unable to accept or hear any possible solutions, I challenge them on this very point. I might say something like: 'I wonder why you are unable to see a positive future? I wonder what that's all about.' It can be tempting to shy away from these kinds of direct conversations, but just like our children mostly do not understand why they behave the way they do, in the same way parents can also get into entrenched patterns of behaviour but haven't stood back and thought about why they think this way.

Section 4: Strategies and solutions

Using *The A–Z* and discussions formed when completing Table 4 in Section 3, the supporter and therapeutic parent can now discuss each behaviour in turn, and plan effective solutions using a strategic approach.

Table 5 is used to formulate a summary and a plan for action, with five questions. Each behaviour should be looked at in turn, although it is likely that there will be similarities emerging across all the behaviours when completing the table.

1. Why might the child be doing what he or she is doing?

The supporter and therapeutic parent should now be able to easily complete this question, using:

- Information from Questions 2, 3 and 5 in Table 4.
- *The A–Z*, behaviour-specific, 'Why it might happen'.
- Knowledge gleaned from discussions during the assessment.
- Discussions with others within the team.

2. Strategies we will use

As the supporter and therapeutic parent look at each behaviour in turn, a good starting point for discussion for appropriate strategies can be found in *The A–Z*. This formulates the basis of discussion and agreement. Where a strategy is suggested that has already been tried and found to be unsuccessful, it is worth revisiting the reasons for this now. Has anything changed? Was it a poor strategy that won't be used again? Might the parent's new perspective have changed the effectiveness of this strategy? Has anything changed around that which now makes it more likely this strategy will be effective? Such as the parent's response?

3. The best time to use these strategies

In order to have the best chance of success, the timing of the implementation of the strategies is critical. If a parent needs back-up, to make sure they can give the child their undivided attention they will need to choose a time when another adult is available.

Other considerations are:

- When the behaviour is most likely to happen.
- What action the child may take (reaction to a new strategy).
- When the parent feels they will be most able to cope.

It is important, however, that the therapeutic parent commits to implementing the strategies as soon as possible, so this should not be seen as an opportunity to introduce delay.

4. What might make this difficult to do? (Obstacles)

Where a difficult behaviour has been experienced over a long period of time, the responses and feelings around it may also have become entrenched. In this question we look at what obstacles might present themselves that will impact on the effectiveness of the implementation of the strategies. Some things to consider are:

- The parent's own feelings. Might they worry about sabotaging the outcome themselves?
- The child taking an unexpected direction. Think of this now. What might it look like?
- Practical issues, such as a second person not being available, or an unexpected event happening.

5. What can we put in place to overcome these obstacles?

As the obstacles have been listed above, the supporter can now assist the parent in planning for success. If it is felt that a second person may not be available, for example, plan for how to ensure that this does not happen. Who can be relied on? Who will the second person be?

Where it has been identified that a child might react in an unexpected way, what does that look like? What will the response be? Make a plan: 'If the child does "a" I will respond "b".'

Once all behaviours have been addressed in turn and strategies agreed, the supporter and therapeutic parent have a plan. They need to be prepared to revisit this plan where necessary. An essential part of the process will therefore be reviewing how things are going – what has worked and what hasn't. At the end of Section 4 a plan to review needs to be made.

PLAN TO REVIEW

The supporter and therapeutic parent must now decide on a time frame to review how well the strategies are working, and to make any necessary changes. It will depend on the nature of the behaviours being tackled as to what form this might take. For example, a behaviour that arises around the ending of school terms would need to be reviewed when there has been an opportunity for that to happen, so the plan to review might be made within 5 days. If the issue is around challenges during transitions, it may be necessary for the problematic transitions to happen several times before an idea of effectiveness can be gleaned.

It may be felt that a review can take place within a few days, but it is likely that a gap of about 1–2 weeks may be needed to properly assess the effectiveness of the strategies implemented.

The supporter and therapeutic parent agree at the end of this section when they will have an interim phone conversation and when they will then meet, the date, time and venue.

In the meantime, the therapeutic parent should also be encouraged to communicate to the supporter any positive or negative changes noted in the child's behaviour.

Visit 5: the review

The purpose of visit 5 is to consolidate, revisit and review progress made. As this whole process has been about 'dousing the sparks', we now need to ensure that the sparks are out, or at least they pose no further threat to stability.

Do not shy away from potential problems but make a note of any new surfacing issues. These can be dealt with later, potentially even within a new BAIRT.

The supporter needs to start this visit by staying focused on the original behavioural issues that were identified within the process. Where strategies have been ineffective, these will surface naturally during the review as Table 2 is revisited and rescored. In order to help the therapeutic parent stay focused, the supporter simply needs to make a note of any new issues arising and reassure them that they will be returning to this.

The review should be positive in tone and remind the therapeutic parent how far they have come, and be a strong visual reminder of progress.

Section 5: Scoring and review

The supporter and therapeutic parent now revisit the scoring that took place in the first visit in Section 1, using Table 2. Referring back to this table, the supporter can record the new scores alongside the original scores. This will help to identify very quickly any improvements and deteriorations, and also to find any new patterns. It is not necessary to dwell for a long time on each behaviour, but simply to quickly record where the parent is in their view of the current behaviours.

Once these scores have been added up, the totals should be inserted into Table 1.

The supporter and therapeutic parent now revisit the scoring that took place in Section 2, Table 3. For this exercise they will use Table 6. This is similar to Table 3, but it is important to record the new scores separately, without being influenced by the original scores. The supporter and therapeutic parent should discuss and think about what has changed and score the *current* severity and perceived impact.

There is likely to be some discussion around how the current behaviours are perceived, what has improved and how the therapeutic parent is feeling. It's important to give time to these discussions, and to allow the conversation to flow naturally. Once the scores have been added up, again the supporter should insert the total into Table 1.

At this point there will be a clear indication of what progress has been made, what has gone well and what needs more work. It can be extremely powerful for both the supporter and the therapeutic parent to see recorded significant changes. Sometimes it may be a very positive surprise and empower the parent further.

IF MORE 'SPARKS' ARE IDENTIFIED

If strategies are found to be failing or are less effective than anticipated, it is essential to revisit Section 3 to double-check that the thinking behind the cause of the behaviours is right. The supporter and parent may wish to involve the rest of the therapeutic team around the child if they feel they are not making progress or if they feel the issues are too complex. In these circumstances it is vital that the team who join these discussions are skilled and knowledgeable in child trauma and therapeutic parenting. Sadly, being a qualified social worker, for example, is no realistic indicator of this unless further post-qualifying training has been undertaken.

THE REVIEW

Once the scoring has taken place, the following eight questions should be deliberated using Table 7. The parent may wish to complete Questions 1–4 themselves, or the supporter can record their words for them if desired.

1. How is the parent feeling about what has happened?

The supporter needs to let the parent take a moment to share their current emotional state and to record this in their own words.

2. What has the therapeutic parent learned about:

a) The child?

It is likely that the therapeutic parent will have gained some insight into the child's thinking and trauma triggers, so record anything that comes to mind here. This is a useful space to look back on, should these behaviours resurface.

b) Therapeutic parenting and child trauma?

Where significant change has been achieved, it's useful to link the therapeutic parenting strategies to changes in behaviours.

c) The agency's practice?

The therapeutic parent should be encouraged to speak honestly and openly about their experiences of the fostering agency and supporter throughout the process.

3. What has changed?

The parent should be able to list here any changes that have occurred. This might be about the behaviours, but is also likely to be about day-to-day life, changes in perceptions, attitudes and thought processes.

4. What still needs to change?

If there are behavioural issues that are still difficult, this needs to be recorded here. It may also be the case that other matters such as school issues or difficulties with the local authority, therapy, short breaks, etc. remain outstanding and need addressing.

5. What has the supporter learned about:

a) The child?
It is likely that the supporter will have gained new insights into the child during this process. These might be similar to those of the parent, or they may be completely different. Sharing these perceptions here enables the parent to look at the changes from different perspectives.

b) The therapeutic parent?
This is an opportunity for the supporter to give the parent positive reinforcement about how they have handled the changes and applied the strategies. The supporter may have discovered new depths of strength, humour and resilience within the therapeutic parent. The parent will be glad to hear these observations.

c) Therapeutic parenting and child trauma?
As this is an equal and joint process, it is important that the supporter shares their own learning with the therapeutic parent. Misunderstandings can arise where a social worker or similar is perceived to be 'the expert'. By sharing joint learning, the supporter and the therapeutic parent break down barriers in their relationship and share knowledge.

d) The agency's practice?
All parties taking part in the assessment should take the time to review what they have learned and if there are learning points for the agency. The supporter may need to be alert to the possibility that they may need to suggest changes to policies and procedures resulting from this assessment.

6. What has changed?
The supporter may use this space to simply summarize the key behavioural changes, but it is a good idea to record changes they have noticed within the attitude and skill of the therapeutic parent, and any changes they have instigated or observed within their own practice.

7. What still needs to change?
If new behaviours have arisen during the process, these need to be recorded here. Similarly, there may be an identification of unmet need for the child and also the parent. This could be the need to provide short breaks in a more structured way, or more support with school.

8. How will this be changed?
The matters that have arisen in Question 6 will determine how this section is answered. For example, if a need for short breaks has been identified, the supporter should record how this need will be met and what steps they will take.

Final discussion

The supporter and therapeutic parent should end the process feeling positive, and at the very least, in a more stable position than at the beginning of the assessment.

Where new issues have arisen, a new BAIRT can be started as part of a pattern of focused, planned visits. This will be especially helpful for practitioners who are unsure about how to proceed and who feel overwhelmed by the complexities of the child's behaviour.

Summary: Implications for Practice

THE TRAUMA TRACKER BY JANE MITCHELL

The Trauma Tracker enables supporting professionals to support the stability of the family because it allows them to examine the presenting behaviours in the context of the child's history. This can enable strategies to be developed that are specific to the child and their history. Crucially this gives the child the relief that someone knows what has happened to them, and the realization that this was not their fault. The parent will be better equipped, the child will have targeted interventions, and the stability of the family will improve.

Using the Trauma Tracker can help the supervising social worker, the attachment therapist and the empathic listener to help the parent to maintain the child's perspective and tie in the child's behaviours with their history, and will inform the Developmental Foundation Planner tool and the Behaviour – Assessment of Impact and Resolution Tool (BAIRT). In addition, the Trauma Tracker gives us a way to place allegations in a historical context and so prevent false allegations and resultant unnecessary disruptions for the child. This is because it identifies past traumatic incidents so that if the child has a trauma memory and makes a false accusation against their parent, which is, in fact, a disclosure, this can be established early on.

DEVELOPMENTAL FOUNDATION PLANNER BY SARAH DILLON

The Developmental Foundation Planner will aid social workers and other supporting professionals to address unmet developmental needs as soon as a child is placed with a family.

This will reduce the number of family breakdowns and unplanned endings because parents and caregivers will learn to effectively respond to a child's developmental and emotional age as opposed to their biological age. It will help supporting professionals to give parents appropriate support and guidance around viewing the child's presenting behaviours as a communication of their unmet needs, which will keep the parent connected to the child through empathic responses, as detailed throughout *The A–Z* (Naish 2018). The practitioner will encourage the parent to focus on what the child is 'saying' to the parent via their behaviour rather than continually becoming embroiled in what the child is 'doing'.

The Developmental Foundation Planner will give supporting professionals the necessary tools to develop their own confidence to become proactive in their approach and in turn reduce the amount of reactionary firefighting we so often see.

THE BEHAVIOUR – ASSESSMENT OF IMPACT AND RESOLUTION TOOL (BAIRT) BY SARAH NAISH

The BAIRT enables practitioners of most levels to engage in an honest, structured process.

At the first signs of 'sparks' (or difficulties), social workers and other trauma specialists can engage on a meaningful level with the therapeutic parent and help them to resolve the issues they face. This means that the relationship between the parent and supporting professional is likely to improve, but crucially, it is *much more* likely that a child will be able to stay in a family, thereby increasing the child's positive chances for:

- Attachment.
- Settled family life.
- Healing from trauma.
- Acceptance of who they are.
- Positive life chances.

The practitioner is likely to feel empowered and more skilled, attaining higher levels of job satisfaction.

After all, why did we become social workers and therapists, if not to improve the lives of others?

References

Brown, B. (2012) *Listening to Shame*. TED Talk.

Gerhardt, S. (2004) *Why Love Matters: How Affection Shapes a Baby's Brain*. New York: Routledge.

Naish, S. (2018) *The A–Z of Therapeutic Parenting: Strategies and Solutions*. London and Philadelphia, PA: Jessica Kingsley Publishers.

Naish, S. and Dillon, S. (2020) *The Quick Guide to Therapeutic Parenting: A Visual Introduction*. London and Philadelphia, PA: Jessica Kingsley Publishers.

Naish, S. and Jefferies, R. (2016) *William Wobbly and the Very Bad Day*. London and Philadelphia, PA: Jessica Kingsley Publishers.

Ottaway, H. and Selwyn, J. (2016) *'No One Told Us It Would Be Like This': Compassion Fatigue and Foster Carers Summary Report*. Bristol: The Hadley Centre, University of Bristol, with Inspire Training Group: Compassion Fatigue and Foster Care. Available at: https://doi.org/10.13140/RG.2.2.33955.45606

Siegel, D.J. (2015) *The Developing Mind: How Relationships and the Brain Interact to Shape Who We Are*. New York: Guilford Press.

The Trauma Tracker Template

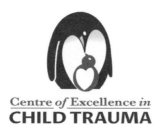

The Trauma Tracker must be used in conjunction with this *Companion*.

Child's name:	Date of birth:	[AQ] Completed by:	Date:
History/chronology	In utero/birth (e.g. domestic violence, drug/alcohol addiction; mental health, illness, birth trauma, premature, maternal illness, abandoned)	Antenatal (e.g. abuse, domestic violence, drug/alcohol addiction, family known to social services; unavailable mother – mental health, addictions, hospitalizations)	Known significant events/dates (e.g. hospitalizations, bereavement, date of removal from family, separation from siblings)

History of family moves (e.g. moves in and out of foster care; kinship care; number of moves, attempted reunification; dates of moves between families)

The impact of these events may be that the child may have strong feelings that families are unsafe

Symptoms of trauma (e.g. generalized anxiety, self-harm, aggression and violence; demand avoidant; stealing, lying, nonsense chatter, attention needing; sexualized behaviours)

Current issues

Potential issues

Event

Links to history

Strategies

Event

Links to history

Strategies

Event

Links to history

Strategies

Event

Links to history

Strategies

The Developmental Foundation Planner Template

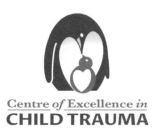

This Planner must be used in conjunction with the Trauma Tracker. It is not designed to be a stand-alone tool. Practitioners using this tool must refer to this *Companion*. Training on the three tools contained within this book can be accessed via the Centre of Excellence in Child Trauma.[1]

Table 1 is generic. For each cornerstone it shows behaviours that can arise from weakness in that cornerstone. As such, it enables the user to identify which behaviours arise from an individual child's unmet developmental needs, and thus which cornerstone needs strengthening first. It is crucial to note that any weakness in Cornerstone 1 must be addressed before any of the others can be successfully tackled. Furthermore, if a child has a deficit in Cornerstone 1, they will definitely have deficits in the other three cornerstones.

---

1 www.coect.co.uk

Table 1. Behaviours that can arise from weaknesses in each cornerstone

Cornerstone 1: Establishing the parent as the unassailable safe base	Cornerstone 2: Developing object permanence	Cornerstone 3: Regular relationship repairs	Cornerstone 4: Linking cause and effect
Avoiding adults to keep safe	Following	Lying	Acting on impulse
Befriending adults to keep safe	Incessant chatter	Stealing	Not considering how their behaviour affects either themselves or other people
Not asking for help	Nonsense questions	Blaming others	Not thinking about the consequence of their behaviour
Fake smiling	Fear of invisibility	Denying responsibility	Inability to project themselves into the future and predict an outcome
Hiding in bedroom	Fear of being forgotten	Defensive rage	Can't learn via punitive consequences, e.g. time out, naughty steps, loss of privileges, being lectured to, etc.
Anxious and clingy	Fear of adult leaving their presence	Controlling and defiant	
Saying that everything is fine when it's not	Frequent need to check availability of adult	Actively but unconsciously seeking rejection, physical punishment, removal of possessions, grounding, loss of privileges, and time out	
Unable to genuinely access adults for comfort and co-regulation	Repeatedly saying 'hello' to an adult when they reappear after a brief absence	Sabotaging birthdays, Christmas and parties	
Not trusting adults to meet their needs	Problems going to sleep	Sabotaging fun	
Innate need to be in control	Frequent waking	Breaking or destroying their belongings, pictures or drawings	
Believing that it is only a matter of time before they are moved on	Calling out in the night	Smearing; urinating in places other than the toilet	
People-pleasing	Difficulty remaining in bedroom	Self-harming	
Rejecting adults	Dysregulation at school	Actively seeking removal from current home	

Lack of sense of belonging	Cannot delay gratification	Irrational anger	
Failing to follow instructions from an adult		Aggressive	
Failing to follow instructions from an adult whilst pretending to do so		Destructive	
Overly compliant			
Secretive			
Withdrawn and insular			
Disingenuous and inauthentic (masking)			
Cannot self-regulate			
Pretending to share the adult's interests			
Aggressive			
Destructive			
Violent			

Table 2 sets out a child's known history and current presenting behaviours. Much of this information can be gathered from the Trauma Tracker.

In Table 2, 'History' means the parts of an individual child's known history that helps to identify their unmet developmental needs. Column 1 contains specific events or experiences and column 2 the consequential unmet developmental needs and associated trauma responses.

Column 3 gives *The A–Z* page reference applicable to column 2, and is only here for the purposes of this book. However, it can be useful to insert the page reference to remind the user where to access the appropriate strategies and solutions necessary to address specific behaviours. Columns 4–7 are for the four cornerstones, and a tick is inserted to indicate where the cornerstone is related to the specific information in column 2.

Once completed, the ticks are tallied up and cornerstones needing the most attention are identified.

Table 2. Child's known history

A	B	Cornerstone 1: Establishing the parent as the unassailable safe base	Cornerstone 2: Developing object permanence	Cornerstone 3: Regular relationship repairs	Cornerstone 4: Linking cause and effect
History/ chronology	Consequential unmet developmental needs and associated trauma responses				
	Total ticks				

After completing Table 2, the user will have a clear picture of how a child's history offers much insight into their unmet developmental needs.

Table 3 looks at current behaviours and identifies the correlating cornerstone. A tick indicates where the cornerstone is related to the behaviours described in column 1.

Table 3. Current presenting behaviours

A	B	Cornerstone 1: Establishing the parent as the unassailable safe base	Cornerstone 2: Developing object permanence	Cornerstone 3: Regular relationship repairs	Cornerstone 4: Linking cause and effect
Current presenting behaviours	*The A–Z behaviour reference page(s)*				
Total ticks					

Completing Tables 2 and 3 enables the user to identify the prioritization of unmet needs. The totals from Tables 2 and 3 are added together to gather an overall total for unmet developmental needs applicable to the cornerstones from a child's known historical chronology and those communicated via behaviour.

The results are then entered into Table 4.

Table 4. Accumulative totals from Tables 2 and 3

Totals	Cornerstone 1	Cornerstone 2	Cornerstone 3	Cornerstone 4
Table 2				
Table 3				
Overall total				

The overall totals give the necessary information for identifying which cornerstones to concentrate on.

Completing Tables 2 and 3 helps to identify the cornerstones in most need of urgent attention, although all cornerstones would also be taken into consideration when planning the necessary approach and strategies for any particular child. This is because, just as in a house, all four cornerstones are needed.

Tables 5–8 can then be completed, one for each cornerstone, in the order of priority (number of ticks in Table 4). Thus Table 5 is for Cornerstone 1 and the user may identify Table 6 for Cornerstone 3 etc. depending on the prioritization of cornerstones in need of strengthening.

In each table, column 1 lists the particular behaviours exhibited by a child under the relevant cornerstones and column 2 details suggested strategies specific to an individual child's needs.

Table 5. Cornerstone 1: Establishing the parent as the unassailable safe base

Exhibited associated behaviours	Suggested strategies from the list in the Developmental Foundation Planner

Table 6. Cornerstone 2: Developing object permanence

Exhibited associated behaviours	Suggested strategies from the list in the Developmental Foundation Planner

Table 7. Cornerstone 3: Regular relationship repairs

Exhibited associated behaviours	Suggested strategies from the list in the Developmental Foundation Planner

Table 8. Cornerstone 4: Linking cause and effect

Exhibited associated behaviours	Suggested strategies from the list in the Developmental Foundation Planner

Table 9 tracks the progress. Column 1 lists the child's presenting behaviours and a tick in column 2 indicates an improvement in these behaviours. Column 3 shows the most useful strategies used by the parent to effect positive change. Column 4 details needs that are being addressed and column 5 suggests actions and strategies for those behaviours yet to improve. Where no action is indicated, the parent is to carry on using the same approach and strategies that have already proved helpful.

Note: 'Improved' doesn't mean the behaviours have dramatically reduced or ceased; it merely shows some improvement, even if only marginal.

Table 9. Progress tracking

Exhibited behaviours	Improved?	Most helpful approach or strategies	Needs being met or addressed	Action or strategies agreed

The Behaviour – Assessment of Impact and Resolution Tool (BAIRT) Template

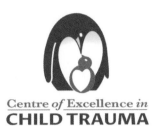

Centre *of* Excellence *in*
CHILD TRAUMA

DEVELOPMENTAL TRAUMA: THE BEHAVIOUR – ASSESSMENT OF IMPACT AND RESOLUTION TOOL (BAIRT)

For full instructions on how to use the BAIRT please refer to this *Companion*. Contact www.coect.co.uk for all associated training.

This assessment tool relies on the assessing supporter and therapeutic parent having access to *The A–Z of Therapeutic Parenting: Strategies and Solutions* (Naish 2018).

Table 1. Comparative scores (front sheet)

Therapeutic parent		
Child		
Supporter		
Date of assessment		
Date of review		
	On first assessment	**On review**
Section 1: Overall behaviour score	Box A	Box D
* Section 2: The three most difficult behaviours score	Box B	Box E
** Section 2: Impact on parent score	Box C	Box F

Notes: * Ensure that the total possible score is also noted, i.e. 3 behaviours will be out of 30, but if only one behaviour is recorded, it will be out of 10.

** As above, note total possible score related to the number of behaviour impacts.

OVERVIEW AND PURPOSE

This questionnaire is designed to assist foster parents, adopters, other therapeutic parents *and* their professional supporters in identifying, understanding and improving or resolving difficult behaviours arising from children who have suffered trauma.

Trauma may be referred to as ACEs (adverse childhood experiences). The cause may be known about, for example, neglect or abuse, or it may stem from an as yet undiscovered event. The important aspect we need to focus on in this assessment is to diminish or resolve the behaviours in order to preserve and promote the evolving attachment between the child and their parent.

The supporter carrying out this assessment should be either a skilled supervising social worker, an empathic listener or therapist (DDP or similar) who is trusted by the parent, and able to feed back progress and seek support themselves from others in the team. Both parties require access to Section 3 in the accompanying *Companion*.

In families where there are two parents, the experience of both may well be different. In some families one parent may feel they are coping well and are not triggered by certain behaviours, while another may feel overwhelmed by a difficult, repetitive behaviour.

The supporter must first identify whom they are working with. Will it be both parents, or just one? If both parents are taking part in the assessment, there will need to be a consensus in Part Two about which behaviours need to be focused on.

No direct work is undertaken with the child other than by the parent.

HOW THE SECTIONS WORK

Section 1: The scope of behaviours. This enables the supporter and parent to work together to establish an overview of any presenting behaviours. It is not necessary to spend a great deal of time looking in depth at each behaviour during the scoring. This section merely allows both parties to start to highlight the areas that the assessment will need to concentrate on.

Section 2: Identifying key behaviours and their impact on the parent. In this section the supporter allows the therapeutic parent the time and space to properly discuss and identify the most difficult behaviours, enabling them to feel heard without blame and judgement. This section is crucial to start to alleviate the effects of compassion fatigue. If the therapeutic parent is in compassion fatigue, they will be unable to hear or implement strategies. The supporter must reduce the stress levels through active, empathic listening without offering solutions, in order to assist the therapeutic parent in accessing empathy for the child and to begin to formulate a strategy. (See *'No One Told Us It Would Be Like This'* [Ottaway and Selwyn 2016].)

Section 3: Analysing three behaviours. This section looks more deeply into each behaviour and analyses where the behaviour might stem from. It is difficult to change or resolve trauma-based behaviours without recognition of *why* they occur. This section also enables the therapeutic parent to reflect on links back to early childhood trauma, and their own triggers. It is possible that a clear and identifiable trigger will emerge. Where an identified trigger is found in Section 3, it is a good idea to resolve this trigger, either through discussion or Havening Techniques, prior to implementing strategies.

Section 4: Strategies and solutions. This section relies on the supporter and therapeutic parent using their pooled knowledge, alongside *The A–Z*, to look at which strategies might work best with the child, and when is the best time to start using them. It is important to make a plan and to be prepared to revisit this plan where necessary. Where strategies are found to fail, it is essential to revisit Section 3 to double-check that the thinking behind the cause of the behaviours is right. The supporter and parent may wish to involve the rest of the therapeutic team around the child if they feel they are not making progress at this point.

Section 5: Review and reflection. It may be felt that a review can take place within a few days, but it is likely that a gap of about 1–2 weeks may be needed to properly assess the effectiveness of the strategies implemented. All parties taking part in the assessment should take the time to review what they have learned and if there are learning points for the fostering agency. The supporter may need to suggest changes to policies and procedures resulting from this assessment.

TIME FRAME

The assessment must be carried out with a supporter, over 2–6 sessions with the therapeutic parents. Where there is a current crisis, the supporter will need to complete

Sections 1 and 2 in the same session and then arrange to start Section 3 within 24 hours. Where the issue is of a less urgent nature, it is possible to do weekly sessions, covering one section per week.

The supporter must remain consistent throughout the assessment and *may not* hand over to another supporting professional midway through, but must put aside the time for the assessment and commit to it. This is to ensure that the therapeutic parent does not have to repeat themselves or loses trust in supporting professionals during a critical process.

Each family will be different, requiring more or less time with their supporter. All parties can complete the table below to help to plan the assessment. As a *minimum*, each assessment should allow the times specified in the 'Recommended timings' column.

Schedule table for this assessment

Section	Recommended timings	Date and time scheduled
Section 1	1–2 hours	
Section 2	2 hours	
Section 3	2 hours	
Section 4	2 hours	
Section 5	1.5 hours	

SECTION 1: THE SCOPE OF BEHAVIOURS

Briefly discuss and score each behaviour:

0 = Not present/no issues

1 = Infrequent, minor issue

2 = Sometimes problematic

3 = Frequent, problematic

4 = Severe, causes/likely to cause big problems

Record the initial behaviour scores in Table 2, column B. (Column C should remain blank at this point in order that it can be completed at the end of the assessment process.)

Table 2. Complete list of behaviours

A	B	C	A	B	C
Behaviour	**Initial score**	**End score**	**Behaviour**	**Initial score**	**End score**
Absconding			Empathy (lack of, child does not care)		
Absences			False allegation		
Aggression (threatening language, etc.)			Fearfulness		
Alcohol			Friendships (difficulties with)		
Anger			Head banging		
Arguing (with adult)			Hiding		
Banging			Hoarding (food or other items)		
Bath time difficulties			Holiday difficulties		
Bedtime issues			Homework		
Bedwetting			Hygiene		
Birthday and other celebrations (reaction to)			Hypervigilant		
Biting			Hypochondria		
Blocking (doorways, etc.)			Immature behaviour		
Boasting			Lateness (being late)		
Brushing teeth (resistance to)			Lying		
Charming (superficial, including fake smile)			Manic laughter		
Chewing			Meal time issues		
Choosing difficulties (unable to make a choice)			Memory issues (forgetfulness)		
Competitiveness (extreme)			Messy bedroom		
Contact (difficult behaviours around)			Moaning/whining		
Controlling			Moving slowly (lagging behind)		
Cruelty to animals			Nonsense chatter/questions		
Damaging items			Obsessive		
Defiance			Over reacting		
Disorganization			Oversensitivity to lights, loud noises, etc.		
Drugs			Poo issues		

A	B	C	A	B	C
Behaviour	**Initial score**	**End score**	**Behaviour**	**Initial score**	**End score**
Racist/sexist etc. behaviour			Social media/phone causing issues		
Refusing to apologize/lack of remorse			Spitting		
Rejecting			Staying in bed (unwilling or unable to get up)		
Rudeness			Stealing (any items excluding food)		
Running off (e.g. in sight, localized running, spur of the moment)			Sugar addiction		
Sabotaging			Swearing		
Separation anxiety			Teasing		
School issues			Throwing things		
Self-harm			Transitions (not managing change)		
Sexualized behaviour			Triangulation (splitting)		
Shouting and/or screaming			Unable to be alone		
Showering			Ungratefulness		
Sibling rivalry			Urinating		
Sleep issues			Violent (actual physical violence)		
Smoking			Additional behaviour (add any not listed)		
Sneakiness					
Total possible	**332**		**Additional scoring**		
Actual total					

Once the totals have been calculated, insert these into Table 1. Use Box A.

SECTION 2: IDENTIFYING KEY BEHAVIOURS AND THEIR IMPACT

Impact on parent: Listening, learning and scoring

The supporter must make an appointment to meet with the therapeutic parent/s in a place where they can speak freely and openly. Sometimes, if time allows and it feels right, this section may flow naturally from Section 1.

Ensure the parent has been given time in a safe, non-judgemental space, to fully explore and explain:

- The impact the child's behaviour has on them.
- Any fears of concerns for self, the child or others.

Identifying key behaviours and their impact

In this section it is important to identify those behaviours that are *most likely* to damage relationship building and/or lead to family breakdown. Use Table 3 to list three behaviours in order of difficulty, 1 being the most difficult (or most pressing issue). Note: If there is only one behaviour, the assessment can continue focusing on just that one aspect.

Table 3. Severity and impact

Behaviour	Severity/frequency	Severity of impact on parent
1	1 2 3 4 5 6 7 8 9 10	1 2 3 4 5 6 7 8 9 10
2	1 2 3 4 5 6 7 8 9 10	1 2 3 4 5 6 7 8 9 10
3	1 2 3 4 5 6 7 8 9 10	1 2 3 4 5 6 7 8 9 10
Totals		

Once the totals have been calculated, insert these into Table 1. Use Box B for severity/frequency of behaviours and Box C for impact on parent.

There must be a break between Sections 2 and 3 where the supporter leaves the therapeutic parent for a minimum of 4 hours, but preferably at least 24 hours. This is to enable both parties to reflect. The therapeutic parent will need recovery time and the supporter will need time and space to ensure the rest of the therapeutic team are aware of progress so far. Advice may also need to be sought from the therapeutic (DDP) lead or other members of the team regarding next steps, analysis and safeguarding.

SECTION 3: ANALYSING THREE BEHAVIOURS

Thinking about each behaviour *in turn*, complete the table below, to see if further understanding can be developed and shared.

Table 4. Analysis of behaviours

	Behaviour 1	Behaviour 2	Behaviour 3
When did it start?			
Was there an obvious trigger? (Think about dates, anniversaries and changes.) If yes, what was the trigger?			
What might the child be communicating through this behaviour?			
Can we identify an unmet need through this behaviour?			
At what age would we normally expect to see this behaviour?			
How does the parent normally respond?			
How might this behaviour link back to early life experiences? (e.g. a child shouting in bed may have been left alone in a cot)			
What strategies have already been tried?			
What happened?			

Parallels and triggers

Can the therapeutic parent think of any parallels from their own childhood or adult emotional experiences that make this particular behaviour especially hard to deal with? If yes, make brief notes.

Notes:

Psycho-sensory therapy session

Where clear triggers are identified within Section 3, sometimes just recognizing those triggers and processing them is all that is required. If these triggers are more problematic, then the supporter can assist the therapeutic parent in accessing psycho-sensory therapies such as mindfulness and Delta Touch Therapies (e.g. Havening Techniques®). This quick and accessible intervention is useful for removing an emotional response to triggering behaviours. If more information is needed, please contact the Centre of Excellence in Child Trauma for recommended referrals.[1]

SECTION 4: STRATEGIES AND SOLUTIONS

Pooling strategies

Using *The A–Z* and the analysis in Section 3, for each behaviour the supporter and therapeutic parent now look at each behaviour in turn to discover and discuss potential strategies.

Table 5. Strategies and solutions

Behaviour 1	
Why might the child be doing what he or she is doing?	
Strategies we will use	
The best time to use these strategies	
What might make this difficult to do? (Obstacles)	
What can we put in place to overcome these obstacles?	

---

1   www.coect.co.uk

Behaviour 2	
Why might the child be doing what he or she is doing?	
Strategies we will use	
The best time to use these strategies	
What might make this difficult to do? (Obstacles)	
What can we put in place to overcome these obstacles?	
Behaviour 3	
Why might the child be doing what he or she is doing?	
Strategies we will use	
The best time to use these strategies	
What might make this difficult to do? (Obstacles)	
What can we put in place to overcome these obstacles?	

Plan to review

The supporter and therapeutic parent must now decide on a time frame to review how well the strategies are working, and to make any necessary changes. It will depend on the nature of the behaviours being tackled as to what form this might take. For example, a behaviour that arises around the ending of school terms would need to be reviewed at that time. Something that happens daily must be reviewed within 5 days.

The supporter will contact the therapeutic parent by phone on . . . . at . . . . to check progress
We will meet to review how well this plan is going on . . . . at . . . .

SECTION 5: REFLECTION AND REVIEW

Revisiting and rescoring

In this section, first the supporter and therapeutic parent will need to revisit and *rescore* *Table 2* in Section 1. The scores must be recorded in column C, 'End score'.

Record the totals for comparison into Table 1 in Box D (on review), on the front sheet.

Now look at Table 3 from Section 2. Think about what has changed and score the *current* severity of both the behaviour and the impact on the therapeutic parent.

Table 6. Rescoring severity and impact

Behaviour	Severity/frequency	Severity of impact on parent
1	1 2 3 4 5 6 7 8 9 10	1 2 3 4 5 6 7 8 9 10
2	1 2 3 4 5 6 7 8 9 10	1 2 3 4 5 6 7 8 9 10
3	1 2 3 4 5 6 7 8 9 10	1 2 3 4 5 6 7 8 9 10
Totals		

Once the totals have been calculated, insert these for comparison into Table 1 on the front sheet. Use Box E (on review), for severity/frequency of behaviours, and Box F (on review), for impact on parent.

Reviewing the process

Now is the time for the supporter and the therapeutic parent to reflect on the process. They should think about what they have learned about each other and how they will use this learning to move forwards.

Table 7. Review

How is the parent feeling about what has happened?	
What has the therapeutic parent learned about: **a) The child?**	
b) Therapeutic parenting and child trauma?	
c) The agency's practice?	

cont.

What has changed?	
What still needs to change?	
What has the supporter learned about: **a) The child?**	
b) The therapeutic parent?	
c) Therapeutic parenting and child trauma?	
d) The agency's practice?	
What has changed?	
What still needs to change?	
How will this be changed?	

Signatures

	Signed	Date
Therapeutic parent		
Therapeutic parent		
Supporter		
Reviewed by line manager/ therapist if appropriate		

Index

A–Z of Therapeutic Parenting, The (Naish) 2, 10
   and BAIRT 97, 99, 100, 110, 121, 124,
      128, 129, 130, 135, 141
   and Developmental Foundation Planner 53,
      54, 55, 56, 57, 58, 59, 65, 66, 69, 70, 72,
      74, 75, 77, 78, 79, 81, 83, 84, 86, 88
   and Trauma Tracker 18, 23, 29, 38
analysing three behaviours in BAIRT
      107–10, 128–35, 164–5
antenatal section of Trauma Tracker 34–6
associated presenting behaviours
   and linking cause and effect 80
   and object permanence 68–9
   and parent as unassailable safe base 63–4
   and regular relationship repairs 73–6
attachment therapists in TRUE model 14

Behaviour – Assessment of Impact and
      Resolution Tool (BAIRT)
   after Trauma Tracker 51–2
   analysing three behaviours 107–10, 128–35, 164–5
   behaviour scoping 102–4, 160–2
   and behaviours from developmental trauma 97–8
   considerations before starting 118
   example of use 100–18
   familiarity with 120
   identifying assessor 119
   identifying behaviours and impact 104–7, 126–31, 163
   parental engagement 119–20
   parental negativity 134–5
   practice implications 142
   and psycho-sensory therapies 132–3, 165
   reflection and review 113–18, 167–8
   review of 136–9
   section outlines of 121–2
   strategies and solutions 110–13, 135–6, 165–6
   template for 157–68
   time frame for completion 101–2, 122–5, 159–60
   time for use 99
   triggers for behaviour 131–2
   uses of 9–11
   workings of 98
behaviour scoping in BAIRT 102–4
behaviours without parent as the
      unassailable safe base 63–4
boundaries for children 65
Brown, B. 57

Centre of Excellence in Child Trauma
      (COECT) 1, 132, 149, 165
child support workers in TRUE model 13

compassion fatigue 75–6
current issues section of Trauma Tracker 43–6

Delta Touch Therapies 24, 165
Delta Wave Therapy 110, 116, 118, 128, 132
Developmental Foundation Planner
   description of 53
   effective use of 59–60
   filling in 81–96
   and four cornerstones of therapeutic parenting 56–8
   linking cause and effect 56–8, 78–81, 92
   object permanence 56–8, 67–73, 93
   parent as the unassailable safe base 56–8, 60–7, 90–1
   regular relationship repairs 56–8, 73–8, 91–2
   template for 149–56
   and unmet developmental needs 54–6, 58–9
   uses of 9–11
   and 'why – what – how' formula of
      children's behaviour 53–4
developmental stages
   early childhood 21–3
   pre-birth 19–21
   in Trauma Tracker 19–23
Dillon, Sarah 17, 30, 36, 45, 51, 67, 134, 141
Dyadic Developmental Psychotherapy (DDP) 13, 98

early childhood development 21–3
empathic commentary
   and object permanence 70
   and therapeutic parenting 66–7
empathetic listening
   in BAIRT 126–7
   in TRUE model 13
encouraging understanding with Trauma Tracker 28

false allegations 24–6
foetal alcohol syndrome (FAS) 20

Gerhardt, Sue 20, 22, 23

Havening Techniques 110, 133, 159, 165
history/chronology section of Trauma Tracker 32–3
history of family moves section of Trauma Tracker 38–41
Hughes, Dan 13

in utero/birth section of Trauma Tracker 34–6

Jefferies, R. 112

known significant events/dates section
    of Trauma Tracker 36–8

linking cause and effect
    associated presenting behaviours 80
    as cornerstone of therapeutic parenting 56–8, 78–81
    description of 78–9
    filling in Developmental Foundation Planner 92
    strategies for 80–1
links to history section of Trauma Tracker 47–9

Naish, Sarah 2
    and BAIRT 97, 100, 112, 131, 134, 157
    and Developmental Foundation Planner 53,
        54, 56, 57, 58, 59, 62, 64, 65, 66, 67, 69,
        70, 72, 73, 74, 75, 76, 77, 79, 81
    and Trauma Tracker 17, 18, 20, 23,
        27, 29, 30, 32, 38, 51, 52
naming the need 67
neonatal abstinence syndrome (NAS) 20

object permanence
    associated presenting behaviours 68–9
    as cornerstone of therapeutic parenting 56–8, 67–73
    description of 67
    empathic commentary 70
    filling in Developmental Foundation Planner 93
    parental presence 69
    responding to needs of child 69
    sleep issues 70–2
    strategies for 69–73
    visual timetables 69
Ottaway, H. 76, 97, 125, 159

Perry, Bruce D. 78–9
play and parent as safe base 66
parent as unassailable safe base
    associated presenting behaviours 63–4
    boundaries for children 65
    'claiming' vocabulary 64
    as cornerstone of therapeutic parenting 56–8, 60–7
    empathic commentary 66–7
    filling in Developmental Foundation Planner 90–1
    giving children own places and things 64
    naming the need 67
    and play 66
    routines for children 65
    self-regulation 64
    strategies for 64–7
    tasks for children 64–5
    visual timetables 65–6
parental negativity 134–5
practice implications
    Behaviour – Assessment of Impact
        and Resolution Tool 142
    Developmental Foundation Planner 141
    Trauma Tracker 141
pre–birth experience
    and developmental stages 19–21
    in Trauma Tracker 19–21
psycho-sensory therapies 132–3, 165

Quick Guide to Therapeutic Parenting, The
    (Naish and Dillon) 67, 134

reactive to proactive practice
    importance of 2–3
    in Trauma Tracker 18
reflection and review of BAIRT 113–18, 167–8
regular relationship repairs
    associated presenting behaviours 73–6
    as cornerstone of therapeutic parenting 56–8, 73–8
    description of 73
    filling in Developmental Foundation Planner 91–2
    reward charts 74–5
    strategies for 76–8
review of BAIRT 136–9
reward charts 74–5
routines for children 65

self-care 52
self-regulation of parents 64
Selwyn, J. 76, 97, 125, 159
Siegel, Daniel 22, 25
significant events section of Trauma Tracker 46–7
sleep issues 70–2
strategies section of Trauma Tracker 49–51
strategies and solutions in BAIRT 110–13, 135–6, 165–6
structures
    and therapeutic parenting 65–6
    and Trauma Tracker 29–30
supervising social workers in TRUE model 13–14
symptoms of trauma section of Trauma Tracker 41–3

tasks for children 64–5
terminology use 11
therapeutic parenting
    description of 2
    four cornerstones of 56–8, 81–96
    linking cause and effect 56–8, 78–81
    object permanence 56–8, 67–73
    parent as the unassailable safe base 56–8, 60–7
    regular relationship repairs 56–8, 73–8
    and Trauma Tracker 23–4
transition difficulties 29
trauma impact 18
Trauma Tracker
    antenatal section of Trauma Tracker 34–6
    background to 17
    case studies 17, 20–1, 24
    client benefits of 15
    current issues section 43–6
    developmental stages in 20–3
    early childhood development 21–3
    encouraging understanding 28
    and false allegations 24–6
    form for 16, 31
    history/chronology section 32–3
    history of family moves section 38–41
    in utero/birth section of Trauma Tracker 34–6
    known significant events/dates section 36–8
    links to history section 47–9
    next steps after 51–2
    overview of 26–7
    practice implications 141

pre–birth experience 19–21
professional use 15
reactive to proactive practice 18
self-care 52
significant events section 46–7
strategies section 49–51
structures in place for 20–30
symptoms of trauma section 41–3
template for 145–7
and therapeutic parenting 23–4
and transition difficulties 29
trauma impact 18
trigger anticipation 27–8
uses of 9–11
triggers
   in BAIRT 131–2
   with Trauma Tracker 27–8

TRUE model
   attachment therapists in 14
   child support workers in 13
   description of 11–14
   empathetic listening 13
   supervising social workers in 13–14
   and Trauma Tracker 32

unmet developmental needs
   and Developmental Foundation Planner 54–6, 58–9
   effects of 58–9

visual timetables 65–6, 69

'why – what – how' formula of children's behaviour 53–4